Conceiving bodies

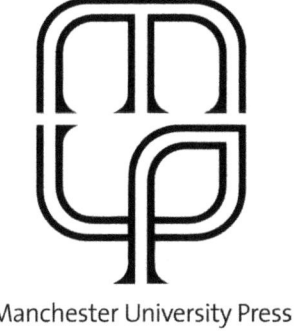

Manchester University Press

MANCHESTER MEDIEVAL LITERATURE AND CULTURE

Series editors: Anke Bernau, David Matthews and James Paz
Series founded by: J. J. Anderson and Gail Ashton
Advisory board: Ruth Evans, Patricia C. Ingham, Andrew James Johnston, Chris Jones, Catherine Karkov, Nicola McDonald, Haruko Momma, Susan Phillips, Sarah Salih, Larry Scanlon, Stephanie Trigg and Matthew Vernon

Manchester Medieval Literature and Culture publishes monographs and essay collections comprising new research informed by current critical methodologies on the literary cultures of the global Middle Ages. We are interested in all periods, from the early Middle Ages through to the late, and we include postmedieval engagements with and representations of the medieval period (or 'medievalism'). 'Literature' is taken in a broad sense, to include the many different medieval genres: imaginative, historical, political, scientific and religious.

This is book 57 in the series. To buy or to find out more about the titles currently available in this series, please go to: https://manchesteruniversitypress.co.uk/series/manchester-medieval-literature-and-culture/

Conceiving bodies

Reproduction in early medieval English medicine

Dana Oswald

MANCHESTER UNIVERSITY PRESS

Copyright © Dana Oswald 2024

The right of Dana Oswald to be identified as the author of this work has been asserted in accordance with the Copyright, Designs and Patents Act 1988.

Published by Manchester University Press
Oxford Road, Manchester, M13 9PL

www.manchesteruniversitypress.co.uk

British Library Cataloguing-in-Publication Data
A catalogue record for this book is available from the British Library

ISBN 978 1 5261 7688 2 hardback

First published 2024

The publisher has no responsibility for the persistence or accuracy of URLs for any external or third-party internet websites referred to in this book, and does not guarantee that any content on such websites is, or will remain, accurate or appropriate.

Typeset by Newgen Publishing UK

For my mother, Linda, and my children, Nola and Leelanau. Thank you for giving me a space to write and something worth writing about.

And for Kath and C. J., who help me see more clearly every time I write.

I dedicate this book to all the women and people who aren't listened to by medical professionals: may their needs be met.

Contents

List of tables	page viii
Preface	ix
Acknowledgements	xii
List of abbreviations	xv

Introduction: Hysteric philology and the occlusion of the ordinary bodies of early medieval English women	1
1 The diagnostic body and the matter of menstruation in the remedies and penitentials	32
2 Fertility and pregnancy in the medical texts and prognostics	68
3 Overlap and overwriting in medical language for childbirth	104
4 Purging as treatment for miscarriage, stillbirth and conception	137
Conclusion: Womb to tomb: The afterlives of early medieval women's remedies	171
Bibliography	192
Index	206

Tables

3.1 Definitions and occurrences of *geberan*,
    cennan, *afedan*, *geeacnian*   *page* 106
3.2 Remedy for wild carrot in *LBIII* and *OEH*   121
3.3 Language in remedies that use *cennan*   124

Preface

I wrote the first draft of Chapter 3 of this book from my basement office, the day after the birthday of my oldest child while in quarantine for the COVID-19 virus in the spring of 2020. Birthdays are a means by which children look forward in time, but by which their parents look back. Most births are scary, if only briefly, but also joyful. This was true of my daughter's birth, and I remember the moment of her birth like a pinpoint. Although I can tell the story of her delivery, I don't remember much of it in the visceral way I remember those moments after it: seeing her as the nurse held her up and thinking at once how long she was, but also 'Oh! She's a *person*.' Her birthday in 2020 brought these postbirth moments back to me, but with a particular sense of gratitude for the historical moment in which she had been born eight years before. People who were pregnant in 2020 did not have the luxuries I had when I gave birth. They were not sure if their partners would be allowed in the delivery room. If they developed the slightest hint of a fever before or after delivery, they knew they would be separated from the babies they gave birth to. If their newborns required the neonatal intensive care unit, they knew that they would lose access to those babies almost entirely until they could be released. The majority of their healthcare personnel were not yet able to be tested for the virus, although they might have had their temperatures checked regularly, not to speak of the vital and grossly undervalued hospital personnel who worked to clean the hospitals and feed the patients. It is in this context that I began my writing about early medieval childbirth, where the paucity of remedies for it is measured against the surplus of remains of women buried during their childbearing years. I suspect the feeling of hopeful expectancy balanced against fearful uncertainty that childbearing people in 2020 experienced is little changed from the long-ago women I study in this book.

My experiences of pregnancy and childbirth are coloured by and colour my work as a scholar. I experience these events as a woman, but there are many ways to be pregnant and to give birth. Trans men and people who identify variously on the spectrum of gender also give birth, and so contemporary experiences of reproductive processes like menstruation and conception are not restricted to women. However, the reproductive body – the conceiving and birth-giving body – of the early Middle Ages was conceptualised as a female body. The social construction of reproduction was reliant upon binary notions of bodies (male and not male), and as such reproductive female bodies were bound by and bound to misogynistic notions of the feminine. My work here centres not on gender and gender expression as fundamental to the category of woman, but rather on the function of the uterus and the specific biological experiences attached to bodies that could give birth.

Just as I have navigated the writing of this book while parenting, so too was the inception of this book inspired by my own experiences of conception, pregnancy and childbirth. Like the medieval women I study, I struggled to conceive (although not because of rickets, thankfully). Like them, I worried through my pregnancy, wishing there was a measure that could tell me that everything inexplicable inside me was progressing safely. My family and friends wrapped me in love and care, just as medieval remedies invoke prayers and incantations for safe and easy conception and birth, and birthing bands encircled the bodies of pregnant medieval women. My hospital birth was nothing like the births these women underwent, and yet the experience was primal, and personal, and in equal parts terrifying and joyful. I was attended mainly by women, and these women occupied all ranks: interns, nurses, midwives and doctors. Yet when I looked to the literary tradition of the time period I studied, I found very few pregnant and birthing women, or women struggling with gynaecological concerns. I found women, yes, and even mothers, but the literary tradition did not think about or represent all those moments that precede the existence of a living child for the woman who must conceive, bear and give birth to that child.

I learned in the process of writing my first book, a book concerned with the bodies of gendered monsters, that the trick to locating sexed and sexualised bodies in Old English literature is to look to unexpected genres. There, I turned to travel narratives and monstrous spaces. In order to find the reproductive bodies of women, I needed to look someplace new, to a genre most often explored to answer questions about efficacy or spiritual belief, about manuscript and textual practices and transmission, or as a part of the history of medicine. I turned to the medical tradition, comprising sets of remedies organised sometimes by malady, but most often by primary ingredient, whether that ingredient be a herb like wild carrot, or parts of various animals, like deer. I learned that this genre relies explicitly on conditions of the body. In the medical tradition, we find descriptions of illnesses and ways of healing those illnesses. Some of those descriptions and remedies for treating bodies feature common-sense elements, and some offer practices that seem not only outlandish and ineffectual, but also inaccessible to ordinary people.

But what the medical tradition does give us are descriptions of women's bodies as they undergo both ordinary and extraordinary reproductive functions. In many ways, this genre is unfazed by the bodies it depicts, contrary to most of the rest of the textual tradition of this time. In other ways, medical texts still struggle with the language necessary to indicate taboo processes and body parts. My work in this book centres on precisely that abjection: women's reproductive bodies that menstruate too much or too little; bodies that swell with life and those that fail to do so; bodies that refuse to remain pregnant, and those that carry on; bodies that give birth, that produce placentas, that require medical purging and social or religious purification. These are the bodies of women, and of people, then and now, who seek care for their troubles, and who turn to the medical tradition to find it.

Acknowledgements

I would like to begin by thanking the University of Wisconsin-Parkside, and especially the College of Arts and Sciences and the Department of Literatures and Languages, for their support of my work, both in terms of course releases and funding, and in terms of intellectual growth and conversation. In a small department, it can be difficult to give faculty members time away from teaching in order to fulfil grants; I'm grateful for the work my colleagues did to offer me this time. My time as a UW-System Fellow with the Institute for Research in the Humanities at the University of Wisconsin-Madison jump-started this project, and allowed me access not only to research materials and time, but to other fellows hard at work on a variety of projects, who read, responded and bolstered my early work on this project. Special thanks go to Jennie Row and Pablo F. Gómez for their insight and generosity.

I cannot offer thanks enough to Bonnie Wheeler and the Dallas Foundation for instituting and maintaining the Bonnie Wheeler Fellowship, and for choosing me as a Bonnie Wheeler Fellow. After COVID-19 decimated my sabbatical, this fellowship provided funding for summer childcare, which allowed me to complete a draft of this book, and to submit it for publication. The Bonnie Wheeler Fellowship is a crucial opportunity for women medievalists with tenure who cannot fulfil the terms of many other fellowships because of familial obligations.

In the process of writing this book, my community of scholarly companions grew significantly, and I'm grateful to each of these people as individuals (too many to name!) as well as to the community of medieval studies scholars who seek fairness and equity in the field. I was welcomed in wholly and treated with great generosity and friendship by Chris Voth, and I am indebted in many ways to her knowledge and collaboration. Robin Norris, Renee Trilling and Rebecca Stephenson helped me to find my community of feminist scholars of medieval medicine in the pages of *Feminist Approaches to Early Medieval England*. I'm glad to be there with Chris and with Erin Sweany, both of whose work inspires me and helps me see these now familiar texts in fresh and exciting ways. I'm deeply honoured to work alongside Lori Ann Garner, and every time I read her work or hear her speak, I am renewed and invigorated in the ways I read and write. Her thorough and immensely helpful commentary on this volume has made it a better, wiser, richer text, and she is in no way responsible for any errors on my part. Thank you to my wonderful editor, Meredith Carroll, at Manchester University Press, who saw the promise in this book many years ago, and who has helped prepare it for the world. Thanks also to Kate Hawkins, Laura Swift, Siobhán Poole and the team at Manchester University Press for their attentive support and the care with which they treated this project. I am particularly grateful for the careful and sensitive reading of Robert Whitelock, who was attentive to and respectful of my American voice, and who caught idiosyncrasies and errors that matter. If this book is about anything, it is about how words matter. It is a delight to work with people who believe the same.

Many thanks to the brilliant artist and also my Wisconsin Women's and Gender Studies Consortium colleague Helen Klebesadel for composing *Natural Healing*, the gorgeous image for the cover of this book. If you look, you'll find the herbal ingredients from the remedies discussed herein: wild carrot, pennyroyal, wallflower, comfrey, blackberry, white dittany and spikenard. She brought to fruition my deepest wishes for the cover of this book, and I am in awe of both her talent and her generosity.

I am incredibly grateful for the friendship and support of my hearth companions, Erin Sweany, Jill Hamilton Clements, Jordan Zweck and Mary Kate Hurley, who are only ever a chat message away, ready to puzzle through a difficult translation; share a necessary file, or a picture of a flower, dog, cat or child; or, via a simple question about citation, find a deeply weird resource on John Clark Hall's beliefs about birth control (thank you, Jordan!). Because of them, and the other wonderful people in these acknowledgements,

I have never felt alone, even though I am the only person in medieval studies at my university.

I am forever grateful to Tom Bredehoft, who helped me find medieval studies via the women in *Beowulf*, and who led me through my first translation of the poem in a long-ago independent study. I miss the insight of Nicholas Howe, who guided me through graduate school, and who made sure that I would have willing friends around to help me, even after he was gone. One of those kind souls is Roy Liuzza, who made sure to say hello at conferences after Nick died, and who pointed me to the prognostics, before I even knew what they were, much less what to do with them.

I could not, and would not, have written this book without the unending support and dialogue of my writing group and dear friends, Kathryn Maude and C. J. Jones. They have read every word on every page of this manuscript more times than I can count. Writing with them is a joy, and my gratitude is deeper than I can say.

I am grateful, above all, to my family and friends. A big thank you goes out to my book group for reading the conclusion, even though it's not as entertaining as a novel; their love of words and stories keeps me fresh and excited to start something new. Robyn Bartlett talked through many a chapter with me on many a walk, and always sends books and soup when we are in need of rescue. My mom's love of books and tolerance for my constant writing helped me find my way as an author; I am grateful to her for never buying me a Nintendo. This book was a labour of love, and it grew alongside my children. They are in every page of this work, and I hope that it participates in a culture that creates greater freedom and bodily autonomy for them.

Finally, thank you to my pups Angus Goodfellow and Zelda Potato, who took me for walks whenever I needed them, but mostly to my partner Drew Carmichael, who has been by my side for two postgraduate degrees; many cats and dogs; two children; and now, two books. I challenge you to another round of *Carcassone*.

Abbreviations

Bald	*Bald's Leechbook*
DOE	Angus Cameron, Ashley Crandell Amos, Antonette diPaolo Healey et al. (eds), *Dictionary of Old English: A to I Online* (Toronto: Dictionary of Old English Project, 2018), https://tapor.library.utoronto.ca/doe/ (accessed 23 December 2023)
DOE Web Corpus	Antoinette diPaolo Healey, with John Price Wilkin and Xin Xiang (eds), *Dictionary of Old English Web Corpus* (Toronto: Dictionary of Old English Project, 2009), https://doe.artsci.utoronto.ca/?p=498 (accessed 23 December 2023)
LBIII	*Leechbook III*
OEH	*Old English Herbarium*
OEM	*Old English Medicina de Quadrupedibus*

Introduction

Hysteric philology and the occlusion of the ordinary bodies of early medieval English women

In Old English medical and prognostic texts, texts engaged in scientific practice and speculation, we have access to the bodies that do not appear in the literary tradition. While most scholarship has read these medical remedies in terms of their efficacy, or as minor contextual agents against which to read other literary texts, I offer instead a literary reading of the remedies. Thinking less about efficacy and more about the embedded beliefs and values these remedies display reveals a perspective on women and their bodies that is absent or overwritten elsewhere in the corpus. The remedies offer a unique opportunity to be in the room with a (perhaps imagined) medieval woman seeking medical help for menstrual woes, or failed conception, or a precarious pregnancy. In fact, the language in these women's remedies is so vague that it is difficult to determine if they intend to treat a woman for infertility or childbirth. Over time, the categories have become hopelessly blurred, perhaps through intentional bias or disavowal, or perhaps through shifting notions of propriety and transgression over time. Translators and scholars have been content to think of these remedies as generally gynaecological, without offering much specific attention to distinctions between the kinds of gynaecological or reproductive concerns a woman might have.

My work in this project dismantles these vague categories by prying apart generalised language and thinking methodically about what each Old English medical term and subset might suggest, not just independently, but systemically. This book unfolds piece by piece the early medieval understanding of menstruation (Chapter 1); fertility and pregnancy (Chapter 2); childbirth

(Chapter 3); and miscarriage, stillbirth, abortion and purging (Chapter 4). In each chapter, I examine the nature of the language as it works to represent the physical lives and experiences of early medieval English women, considering both the absences and presences in the textual tradition, and arguing for the specific ways in which women both did and did not exert agency over their own bodies and reproductive identities.

This introduction establishes the foundations necessary for understanding medical texts in a number of different and parallel frameworks: practices of language, the textual and manuscript tradition of medicine in general and women's medicine specifically, the practices of later translators and dictionary-writers, and the physical experience of women's lives in early medieval England relative to the dangers of reproduction. Each of these pieces is essential groundwork for thinking about how early medieval English remedies for women function, and why these functions matter for the ways we think about the extraordinary bodies of ordinary women.

The Old English medical tradition and the present absence of women's medicine

Medieval medical texts are generally constructed as collections of medical treatments for a variety of human ailments, both ordinary and extraordinary. Some of the collections are organised around the ingredients they require, while others are structured around the malady they treat. For instance, *Leechbook III* begins with eight treatments for headache, varying from the use of mustard, rue and pennyroyal to small stones from the mouths of young swallows, for the express purpose of addressing 'nihtgengan' ('night-goers').[1] The headache remedies are immediately followed by treatments for swollen eyes that include remedies made of such ingredients as the eyes of live crabs, children's urine, 'suet of a fox' and honey.[2] Alternatively, the *Old English Herbarium* begins with twenty-nine remedies using *betonica* (wood bettany) for ailments that include a 'shattered skull', 'watery eyes', 'pain in the loins', 'blood gushing through the mouth', 'not getting drunk', 'feeling unwell or nauseous' and snakebite.[3] One needn't look hard to find remedies that are strange or shock-provoking. All too often, the remedies are overlooked as serious or important texts because of these perceived qualities. And yet the remedies reveal much about the culture that recorded and potentially made use of them, beyond whether they worked or not.

The medical texts typically begin with tables of contents that precede the remedies themselves. One of my favourite mysteries in the Old English medical tradition centres on *Bald's Leechbook* (*Bald*),[4] which offers a 'Table of Contents' prior to sharing its 1,139 remedies. In this case, the 'Table of Contents' indicates where to find remedies for which maladies, but also identifies remedies that are now missing from the main text. The remedies that are missing? As Christine Voth notes in her dissertation: 'The chapters with the highest remedy counts are those that are, sadly, missing, including forty-one obstetric treatments and seventy-five for the treatment of diarrhoea and dysentery.'[5] While all those remedies for stomach and bowel ailments might have contributed to our understanding of those illnesses, *Bald* still features an entire chapter (Chapter 30) in which he shares further remedies for similar ailments. He includes no other remedies for women's medicine. The 'Table of Contents' cannot tell us why those remedies are missing – through accident or by some censorial hand – but it reveals to us that such remedies were once included as part of this text, that they merited a specific section and that they no longer exist.[6] The mystery of these remedies is sometimes frustrating: what might they have told us about women's medicine that the other existing remedies in the tradition do not? Where might they have confirmed a principal treatment or offered a variation or detail? But the mystery, and the fundamental unknowability to which it is attached, is at the heart of the medical treatment of women's reproductive bodies. In order to study this field, there are so many questions we cannot answer. Were the medical texts used widely to treat real people with real ailments? Were there local practitioners who helped those suffering with illnesses? Was there a tradition of medical practices that circulated outside the literate and textual traditions? In truth, we can never answer these questions with certainty. We are limited by a finite number of texts and a historical moment in which literacy was similarly limited.[7] It seems that we have more mysteries about what these texts comprised and how they were used than we have answers.

This is not to say that there is a shortage of important and vibrant analyses of the medical tradition, arguing vigorously against long-held and stereotypical visions of early medieval medicine as primitive and laughable. Early medieval English medical practice has benefited from recent nuanced work that moves past dismissive preconceptions. Monica Green's work on medieval women's medicine serves as a touchstone for this book, and Christina Lee's AncientBiotics project works collaboratively to identify and study potential contemporary use of medieval medical practices and compounds.[8] As Christine Voth has noted, the work of many contemporary women scholars has 'brought the subject into the modern field of the history of medicine'.[9] These works stand in conversation with a long history of disdain and shock at the perceived strangeness of early practice. Even as late as 2007, David Wootton suggested that early medieval English texts are universally accepted to be 'bad medicine', echoed two years later by Peregrine Horden's pronouncement, 'Let us concede that early medieval medicine did not work.'[10] Horden's point was that rather than focusing on biomedical efficacy, we should consider patients' beliefs regarding their treatment, 'allowing for more complexity beyond whether a treatment works or not (most commonly not)'.[11] Often contemporary readers use these ideas to focus on magic and superstition, without proper grounding in the systems of belief Horden references. Similarly, Rebecca Brackmann's work encourages the reconsideration of the placebo effect as a useful and productive medical mechanism, which should disrupt our presentist assumptions about medical efficacy in the Middle Ages, and Erin Sweany urges caution in the cross-cultural comparison of the Old English corpus of medical texts, suggesting that 'we must be careful not to exploit the medical corpora of other cultures for the sake of Eurocentric insights'.[12] These sophisticated contemporary readings work to move us away from shock at often startling early medieval medical practices, and ask us to think instead about the complex cultural motivations and systems at work in and foundational to the Old English medical corpus.

Much needed new editions of the early English medical texts, recently published and forthcoming from Dumbarton Oaks, signal a rising interest in and attention to these important works. Our understanding of early medieval English medicine comes primarily from five texts: *Bald*, *Leechbook III* (*LBIII*), the *Lacnunga*, the *Old English Herbarium* (*OEH*) and the *Old English Medicina de Quadrupedibus* (*OEM*).[13] Both *Bald* and *LBIII* are in a single, shared manuscript, London, British Library, Royal 12.D.xvii. London, British Library, Harley 585 includes the *Lacnunga* as well as *OEH* and *OEM*, and the last of these texts also occurs in three additional manuscripts.[14] *Bald* seems to have a strong Mediterranean influence, and 'contains an impressively wide-ranging collection of remedies, as well as sections of careful and sustained discussion drawn from Late Antique medical compendia'.[15] *LBIII* seems to offer northern European traditions, often associated with 'native' as opposed to 'learned', although many of these remedies have their foundations in Pliny. *Lacnunga* similarly features remedies that have been associated with magic and superstition, although Kesling successfully counters previous understandings and locates these remedies solidly in the Hiberno-Latin tradition. Featured as they are in multiple manuscripts, *OEH* and *OEM* were probably produced in a highly learned context, with strong connections to continental sources.[16]

The learned tradition seems to have derived from a tradition both literate and oral, situated in Benedictine monasteries, and drawing on Latin and Byzantine traditions including Pliny, Dioscorides and Galen. Anne Van Arsdall notes that:

> not only were medical texts ... copied, excerpted, and used as references by monks who treated sick people, but the monks and infirmaries were also a source for medical information on healing, on medicines, and on growing and collecting medicinal herbs. This knowledge was passed orally and in written form from monks to other monks, to patients and to lay persons.[17]

Thus, monasteries were the spaces in which texts were created, recreated and shared, but they were also a location in which remedies might be adapted or added based on actual practices. Indeed, the translation of such texts as the *OEH* from Latin into the vernacular suggests the use value of the text by practitioners, particularly since we have multiple manuscript versions of the translation.[18] Kesling argues that despite their current marginal positioning in the literary tradition, medical texts held an 'important place in Anglo-Saxon libraries ... [they] were also among the genres of text most chosen for translation, even if translation in this field would have required special expertise'.[19] The textual tradition, then, is bound up with a particular kind of practice and practitioner: expert and learned practitioners affiliated with monastery systems.[20]

The nature of the texts themselves offers some help in determining who might have practised medicine in England in the early Middle Ages, although these texts privilege only certain kinds of literate medical practitioners. Some scholars claim that the need for translations from the Latin indicates that not all practitioners would have been religious. M. L. Cameron, for example, suggests that laymen also seem to have practised medicine:

> If laymen were physicians, they must have been reasonably well educated, as surviving medical documents draw generously on Latin medical texts and give ample evidence that they were intended to be manuals for practicing physicians and that they were so used. Perhaps it was because lay physicians could not be expected to be proficient in Latin that there was so much translation from Latin medical works into English. But there is equally good evidence that physicians were members of religious orders.[21]

The consensus around medical texts suggests that learned practitioners were mostly male, although not exclusively themselves celibate or attached exclusively to positions inside religious institutions.[22] However, Fiona Stoertz suggests that monks, 'in spite of the medical function of monasteries as infirmaries in the early Middle Ages, probably had no practical experience of birth'.[23] She argues instead that birthing women likely were attended almost exclusively by women whose literacy and access to such texts is extremely unlikely. The medical books are written by and for men, and they rarely make mention of women as healers or reference the presence of midwives.

In the case of women's medicine, we are faced with the strong temptation to invent a practitioner who does not exist in the textual tradition: the village midwife. Indeed, the word for midwife in Old English, *byrþþinen*, or *beorþorþinen*, occurs only thrice in the corpus, which might suggest the relative unimportance of such a figure, or the erasure of it.[24] Cameron argues that it is extremely unlikely that women healers did not exist: 'Surely there were women midwives and village women gatherers of herbs and wise in their use and women learned in charms and amulets. But there is not a shred of evidence for their existence.'[25] However, in 'Gendering Women's Health Care', Green counters the fetishised idea of the 'golden age' of women's healthcare, in which women did and knew everything, a fantasy that hinges on the figure of the witch-midwife as a figure of persecution and desire for control.[26] Green argues not that women did not attend births, but rather that 'women's routine attendance at normal childbirth was not threatened because this was not normally seen as a "medical" condition that demanded the physician's or surgeon's intervention'.[27] We can read Green's argument in two ways: (1) women were not the primary practitioners responsible for women's medicine, particularly with respect to medicine represented in the textual tradition; but also (2) women *did* attend women in childbirth and presumably for other ordinary gynaecological questions or needs, but these needs might not have been understood as particularly 'medical'. Thus, it seems likely that there was a community of women sharing personal, if not what Green would consider professional, knowledge, but that that knowledge is neither part of nor represented in the literate medical tradition.

If women practitioners are absent from the medical corpora, women's medicine is not – at least not entirely. As the missing section of *Bald* that I discussed above suggests, remedies for women's reproductive maladies were part of the tradition, and even though that specific subset of remedies is missing, women's remedies remain in other texts. The percentage of women's remedies relative to the corpus as a whole is very small, and many parts of it seem to be missing. In her doctoral thesis, Emily Kesling suggests:

> Of 25 remedies omitted out of the first 100 chapters of the *Herbarium*, at least 4 pertain specifically to women. This count far exceeds the normal proportion of remedies specifically related to women in the *Old English Herbarium*, whose first 100 chapters, divided into approximately 350 individual remedies, contain only 8 cures specifically related to women.[28]

Thus, remedies for women are rare, and even despite that rarity, existing remedies for women's maladies seem to have been omitted from the textual tradition through a variety of mechanisms.

Determining the actual number of existing remedies for women is complicated: in a search of the *Dictionary of Old English Web Corpus* (hereafter *DOE Web Corpus*), the word *wif* occurs 111 times across all of the possible remedies, but these occurrences do not even reflect the number of remedies specific to women, as often *wif* occurs multiple times in a single remedy, and sometimes *wif* is used to modify the word milk, as breastmilk was an occasional ingredient in general remedies.[29] Further, the medical texts are often structured with a table of contents that indicates the contents of actual chapters, and so phrases and types of remedies are repeated, if we search only for language. There is no real shortcut to locating women's remedies, although language can help us find them. But a true count of gynaecological remedies reveals the following numbers: *Bald*: forty-one missing remedies with thirteen specific ailments listed in the 'Table of Contents'; *LBIII*: eight remedies; *Lacnunga*: three remedies; *OEH*: twenty-two remedies; *OEM*: fourteen remedies. These manuscripts include other remedies that might apply to women, including remedies for breast or chest pain (like *OEM* 19.3, which addresses nipple pain for nursing women), and for arousing desire for sexual intercourse (for example *OEM* 6.11, which makes use of goat's gall and nettle to increase pleasure for women).[30] If we count generously, the medical texts include eighty-eight remedies specific to gynaecological concerns. If we leave out the missing remedies from *Bald*, we are left with only forty-seven gynaecological remedies. Thus, assuming there are thousands of remedies in total (extrapolating from Voth's count of 1,139 in *Bald* alone), approximately 1 per cent of Old English remedies address the concerns of women. Considering the fact that many women died as a result of reproductive complications at this time, this percentage is bleak, even if we consider that other remedies for women might have existed, but have been lost.

However, even if we did have access to all possible remedies for women, the remedies are a cipher. They reveal *something* about medieval medicine and bodies and practices, but what is it that they reveal, beyond how medicine may have been practised on actual medieval bodies? They reveal beliefs about bodies, beliefs informed by earlier traditions and by the religious status of the scribes and compilers of such manuscripts; about practices that might or might not be taking place in monasteries serving as infirmaries; about cultural practices of exclusion and abjection.[31] They are a record of some forms of belief about women's bodies, providing at once evidence of men's beliefs about women's bodies *and* evidence of women's bodies. That is, they offer representations of actual, and not exceptional, early medieval English women, in the sense that we normally find women present in the tradition to be exceptional.[32] However, the concerns of the women as reflected by remedies are both ordinary, in their implied ubiquity, and extraordinary, in what they reveal about women's possible control over their own bodies.

The effacement of everyday women

Access to women's bodies is limited by the very structure of the early medieval literary tradition – a tradition defined by and delimited by men. In *Double Agents* (2001), Clare Lees and Gillian Overing argued that since we very often cannot find early medieval women in the literary tradition, we should look for vestiges of them in silences and spaces of absence.[33] The bodies of ordinary women rarely appear in Old English texts. Literary women are exceptional: saints, queens and even monsters. For example, *Beowulf* features seven women, all of whom are of high status (or a lone monster), but only one of these women actually speaks in the text: the queen, Wealhtheow. Not only do we not hear from these other six women, we never even see lower-status women at all – no one cooking, or sweeping, or taking care of the children. The same is generally true across the corpus: the women who appear in texts are the highest of high-status figures: queens like Emma, stateswomen like Æþelflæd, abbesses like Hild, saints like Juliana or Elene, religious matriarchs from Eve to Mary. Few women speak in the corpus, and if they do, they do so from a lofty social position. As a result, the literary tradition reveals little to us of the experience of ordinary women, the women not married to prestigious men, or themselves leaders of religious orders. When the women in the tradition do speak, their discourse is rarely centred on the body: instead they participate in statecraft or the development of religious practices. We find little in this textual tradition to reveal the daily lives of women, whether of high or low status, and even less about their reproductive bodies beyond the children they produce.

Where the literary tradition is limited in its representation of women's reproductive bodies, archaeology has access to both the bodies of women and material objects connected to their identities. The remains of medieval women provide evidence of the physiological processes that informed their lives and their deaths. And yet, despite the comparative wealth of archaeological evidence, close examination of women's bodies in graves often reveals a continuation of the focus on high-status women. The evidence of such graves must necessarily skew understanding of the experiences of all women; what is true for high-status women in terms of nutrition and physical conditions is not necessarily universally true for women living in very different circumstances. Gale Owen-Crocker explains:

> Although we have their bones and we have their teeth, the evidence about the lives of these women from pathology is very small. They were generally well nourished, with no dental decay and an adequate supply of protein in their diet; or at least the women who had sufficient status to be buried in the cemetery were. There are clearly fewer documented burials than there were Anglo-Saxons and we do not know what happened to the results of deformity at birth, poverty, and starvation: tossed into the river, dumped into the wood?[34]

Like the literary tradition, often graveyards reveal the experiences of high-status women, once again standing in for, and perhaps even concealing the experience of, ordinary women. The work of Duncan Sayer and Sam D. Dickinson does examine women from a range of social classes in its discussion of double graves. They suggest that 'these were not special burials but women from the whole social spectrum, and women who worked'.[35] Certainly not all graves are universally reserved for the wealthy, but as with so much of early medieval English material, much has been lost, and we are left to make assumptions based on the evidence that remains. Further, interpretation of this data, particularly with respect to women's bodies, has often been underexamined or read only in terms of existing expectations.

In this way, graveyards seem to explain what the textual tradition does not: that childbirth was a dangerous event for early medieval women. Sally Crawford observes:

> at the fifth- to seventh-century cemetery site at Berinsfield, Oxfordshire, adult female deaths below the age of thirty were considerably greater than those of males in the same age group … At the late [Anglo-Saxon] rural church cemetery of Raunds, Northamptonshire, 44 per cent of all adult females died between the ages of seventeen and twenty-five, that is, during their optimal period of childbearing.[36]

These numbers reveal that women died most frequently at the ages during which they would have been most fertile. Sayer and Dickinson claim that 'maternal mortality … may have been the cause of up to 50% of young female fatalities and is the cause of 30–40 per cent of death in the modern developing world';[37] they examine graves shared by women and foetuses or infants, debunking the notion of 'coffin births', where a pregnant woman was buried and seemed to have given birth post mortem. Instead they suggest a complex range of burial practices that attempt to mark the relationship between women and infants, indicating death in, and as a later result of, childbirth. Caroline Batten suggests that 'these various arrangements of women with fetuses and neonates represent a kind of entangled death: such burials not only visually mark labor as the cause of death, highlighting its particular danger, but also seem to blur the identities of mother and child'.[38] These rare double burials, however, cannot represent all deaths that occur as a result of childbirth. Sayer and Dickinson argue against the conservative estimations of Calvin Wells, who 'was certain that the only way to identify death in childbirth was by direct association, where the foetus is found in the pelvic canal'.[39] Using only this metric to determine maternal mortality probably underrepresents actual percentages significantly, and distorts the experiences of early medieval women giving birth.

In cases less obvious than intertwined births, a woman's age at death has been the primary metric used to determine the cause of her mortality, even when other measures might reveal a more complex narrative. The scholarly tradition has been content, generally, to assume that childbirth is the cause of death for women in these age ranges; this simplified explanation has been perceived as satisfying enough, meriting little further investigation. But accepting this simplification about women's deaths is an integral element in the long history of experts misreading or overlooking evidence about women's bodies. Recent scholarship, like that of Sayer and Dickinson, works to counter these assumptions through thoughtful considerations of mortuary evidence and burial practices; they suggest that 'we will never know how many, or which, women died in childbirth but, as maternal death is a significant factor in patterns of female mortality, we may get an impression of its extent from comparative mortuary demographics'.[40] Indeed, devoting resources to the study of women's bodies may yield important clarification. Owen-Crocker argues that 'Forensic archaeology offers important ways forward for Anglo-Saxon cultural studies. Testing for the amount of collagen in bones apparently indicates pregnancy or lactation. The assumption that 20s–30s death rates were related to childbirth could be tested by these means.'[41] Certain kinds of testing might offer us more nuanced information about the causes of death of the existing remains.

Without such testing, and perhaps even with it, we cannot determine what parts of the reproductive process might have caused women's deaths – haemorrhage, sepsis, eclampsia, infection or post-delivery haemorrhage might well have killed women up to forty-two days postpartum.[42] All too often, the scholarly tradition has been content to accept the broad parameters of this category – maternal mortality. Part of this acceptance is through exigence: we cannot determine answers based on the data that remains or with the limitations of funding for certain kinds of research. Part, however, reveals a larger cultural incuriosity; all the elements of reproductive danger are tidily lumped together. What if death in childbirth is not the primary culprit in women's deaths? What if early pregnancy or other mechanisms for ending pregnancy are also causes? It is not enough to be content that 'reproduction' causes death; we should want to know which reproductive processes endangered the lives of women, because those reproductive causes *still* endanger the lives of women today.

Therefore, while archaeology provides access to the physical experiences of early medieval women, the study of these remains is also characterised by lack: lack of remains that represent the entire range of social experiences; lack of soft tissue that can reveal important information about disease or pathology; lack of adequate funds for testing, or even value for the testing of certain kinds of bodies. What archaeology does reveal is that reproductive causes seem to underlie the deaths of many, many women. Sayer and Dickinson suggest that 'Everyone would have known someone who had, or would, die in childbirth.'[43] Maternal mortality seems to have been rampant, and dangers to both mother and child are significant. And yet the shockingly low proportion of remedies – efficacious or not – for women's crises of fertility and childbirth reveals a textual medical tradition that demonstrates very little care for or attention to the bodies of women.

Medieval remedies for reproductive processes exist, and yet determining their functions is complicated by occlusion around the language for women's bodies. There is no Old English word for womb. The Old English word *wamb* means not womb, as we conceive of the location in which a foetus resides, but rather 'belly, stomach'.[44] When Old English medical texts refer to pain in the womb, they refer to the bodies of both men and women. Religious texts tend to use *innoðe*, a word that the Bosworth–Toller Old English Dictionary defines as 'the inner part of the body'; 'stomach, womb, belly'; a place referred to in relation to feelings or emotions, as well as the seat of appetite, or even 'entrails'.[45] Similarly, there is no specific Old English term for vagina (notably, a word that means, in Latin, 'sheath', or 'sword-holder'; the corresponding term in Old English, *sceað*, is not used to indicate this body part). Men's and women's reproductive organs are grouped generally under the term (and its variants) *gecynd* or *cennende*, terms so general that they hold a range of meanings from parent to kind/genus. While the *Thesaurus of Old English* offers five possible terms used for penis (*lim, pintel, scamlim, teors, wæpen*),[46] no such matches occur for vagina, womb or even pudenda. A range of terms show up as glosses for *matrix*, but do not occur in texts as references to the uterus.[47] The closest I have found is the term *gecyndlim*, 'birth-limb, womb, vulva', a term that occurs twelve times in the corpus of Old English writing, and which can also mean 'sexual organs. 1. Of a male, genitalia'.[48] The medical texts simply do not use discrete language to describe the uterus in any sort of specific way. This absence of naming does not necessarily mean that women's bodies did not matter in early medicine, but identifying the parts of these bodies specific to women seems not to have mattered.

The problem with this occlusion of bodies and of naming is that, in the medical texts, discrete names for women's reproductive body parts and processes are either absent or obscured through the vicissitudes of language and a squeamish scholarly tradition that finds women's bodies either distasteful or unworthy of attention. The names of the elements of women's bodies, in true Galenic fashion, are simply variations on the names for elements of men's bodies.[49] The medical texts rely on a system that groups all bodies into a single gender category, *mann* – a term that means person, but which I argue suggests 'man' as the default person – or specifically indicate that certain remedies, rarely, are meant for female bodies. The male body is the standard, the default, the universal. All bodies are understood to be variations of that single (male) body.

In this book, I use the language employed by the medical texts, which relies on a gender binary of male/female and man/woman. The remedies use this language, but I do not wish to suggest that this binary is either real or universal, even in the Middle Ages: Leah DeVun argues that in Latin Europe, 'the important difference between male and female was a matter of continuity and degree, rather than of bipolar distinction'.[50] Through thinking about the nature of bodies identified as female, we can make space in the scholarly tradition for a range identities and genders beyond the default of the idealised male form. However, bodies with female organs do not function in the same ways that bodies with male organs do, and often do not experience illness in the same ways that male bodies do. If treatments presume that female bodies are faulty male bodies, then 'health' will be sought by suppressing female organs rather than facilitating their function.

Hysteric philology: Building an intersectional feminist methodology

Because women's bodies are effaced from the larger critical tradition through a variety of mechanisms, we must examine the tools and methods that participate in this effacement. In truth, women's bodies are *not* absent; they are in graves, in sculpted forms and in the medical texts. The biggest impediment in the search for early medieval English women's medicine is the assumption that there is little to find; the lack of clear language around women's remedies is one of the ways in which dictionaries and editions perpetuate this problem.

It is difficult to determine how many remedies there are for women's maladies because the tools for reading these texts participate in their obfuscation: as a result of translations and dictionaries, all gynaecological illness is lumped together as 'women's problems', and because these remedies are rare and often oblique, the scholarly conversation implicitly dismisses them as unworthy of extended attention. The discipline of Old English studies is balanced between the nineteenth-century tools, editions and translations, and a mindful contemporary praxis of traditional methodologies, even as it negotiates its own naming. As Mary Rambaran-Olm has rightly argued, 'the truth is that our field was founded on white supremacy', noting the systems social, political and academic that depended and depend still on racist ideologies.[51] Adam Miyashiro has been integral in the critique of the racist and sexist epistemes of the nineteenth century as well as of the present moment, critiquing the very tools scholars use as embedded in a carrying forward of forms of white supremacy and sexist and racist ideas.[52]

Tools like the Bosworth–Toller *Anglo-Saxon Dictionary* and many of the volumes produced by the Early English Text Society (EETS) provide the only access and interpretation available to many scholars of Old English. These tools and editions efface and misrepresent content in the texts that they find objectionable or challenging, and scholars often have no choice but to trust the textual tradition as it is perpetuated through these resources. For many years, scholars have treated these materials as truths, and accepted what they say about medicine. Both T. O. Cockayne's use of Latin to describe female bodies rather than offering a translation into English, and the continued scholarly use of dictionaries composed originally in the nineteenth century to describe women's maladies in figurative ways, result in the compression and generalisation of women's medicine. All the remedies for women fit together nicely in the capacious category of 'women's medicine', without very much thought or attention devoted to the limits and distinctions that exist inside this category.

It is no surprise that nineteenth-century men's approaches to women's medicine might be problematic. And yet their methods, and particularly philology, remain at the heart of the field of Old English studies. These men created the research tools upon which this discipline relies; theirs are the tools most readily available to scholars without institutional access to research libraries. In using their methods and their tools, it can be difficult for contemporary scholars to recognise the kinds of harm and indeed the limits such tools place on the texts we seek to examine. This does not mean we should reject philology, or even the Bosworth–Toller dictionary – a tool I use consistently in both my teaching and in my research for this book. But we must be careful about the ways we use these tools, and, indeed, about the ways we use philology. The limitations of these existing tools require not the end of philology, but rather more, and more thoughtful, philology.

In my own examination of the medical texts, I have learned that effacement of women results not just from the original author's unconcern with women's remedies, or even nineteenth-century discomfort with women's bodies. Instead, much of the harm comes from contemporary scholars adopting these approaches at face value. In the scholarship, frequently women's remedies are grouped as generally 'reproductive'. I started to ask why, and what I found was that the language was so obscure, so figurative, so frustratingly inconclusive, that it became simpler to unify these remedies as a singular category – women's medicine – without thinking much more about them. But when I started to look more closely, what I found was that the language looked like this not only because of its own occlusiveness, but because of the layers of wallpaper that had been laid upon it. The dictionaries, the editions, the contemporary essays, even the University of Toronto's *Dictionary of Old English*, perpetuated the idea that the terms could not be specified. But, with careful attention to the specific occurrences in the remedies themselves, and by virtue of these remedies' relation with one another, I engage in a new kind of philology, one that uses the old tools enthusiastically but also with suspicion. I work to understand the discrete language around women's bodies, and to think through the different kinds of maladies that are raised and treated in the medical tradition.

While calling in the tools of the discipline makes a space for voices and identities that have been omitted from the scholarly tradition, another part of my methodology calls for grounding in the contemporary moment. The bodies of women in the past are informed by their social and historical context, and this context matters deeply, but the bodies of those women matter in the contemporary moment because of the reproductive bodies of people today. If I write about medieval childbirth, then I also must think about modern childbirth. If I study the many women who died in the early Middle Ages as a result of reproductive problems and the nutritional deficits that both preceded and resulted from childbirth, then I also need to think about women now who still die in childbirth. Black and Indigenous women in America are 'two to three times more likely to die from pregnancy-related causes than white women', even among women with the highest levels of education.[53] The National Black Women's Reproductive Justice Agenda places this percentage more precisely for Black women, indicating that they are 3.5 times more likely to die from pregnancy complications than white women in the United States of America, while they are more likely to experience unintended pregnancies, and to experience sexually transmitted diseases, as well as being twice as likely to die of cervical cancer – problems significantly exacerbated by the fact that Black women are 55 per cent more likely to be uninsured than white women.[54] Deirdre Cooper Owens explores the long history of Black women's medicine in America, wherein in 1865, Black women were described as possessing 'near immunity from pain during childbirth', a belief that resulted in the gross mistreatment of Black women in terms of research over many generations, and which has resulted in a current set of stereotypical and fictional beliefs held by white medical students about 'Black people's alleged biological differences from white people'.[55] These beliefs about the differences between Black women and white women inform the consistent dismissal of Black women's voices as they advocate for their own medical health and safety.

Not only does contemporary medicine fail Black and Indigenous women as they give birth, but it fails all women in flawed methods of research that are informed by the familiar medieval belief in a universal (read: white, cis, able, male) body. Contemporary medical systems from research to individual practice to financial support fail women and people with uteruses in serious ways. It is commonplace to suggest that medieval medicine failed women, but modern medicine is not doing much better. According to Imogen Learmonth, 'Learning from male bodies is frequently the default in clinical trials today, where subjects are overwhelmingly men – even the standard laboratory mice are male.'[56] Women's heart attacks, which often feature different symptoms than men's, have not been well understood, leading to thousands of women self-reporting concerns of dying of heart attacks without being taken seriously by their physicians.

Research funding for women's medicine is abysmal, with funding for erectile dysfunction receiving five times more funding than research into endometriosis. Indeed, according to Learmonth, 'less than 2.5% of publicly funded research has been dedicated exclusively to female reproductive health despite the fact that one third of women will experience severe reproductive health issues in their lifetime'.[57] Nicola Slawson, too, cites the disproportion of research funding for women's medicine relative to men's, a problem that virtually steps out of the pages of early medieval medicine: 'There is five times more research into erectile dysfunction, which affects 19% of men, than into premenstrual syndrome, which affects 90% of women.'[58] Contemporary medicine continues to bear these assumptions about which bodies are universal, and which are deviant; which bodies function as the default, and which require special consideration. Modern medicine, like medieval medicine, fetishises default bodies that do not represent the actual population. It neglects bodies that do not abide by the limits of the default – white, male, cis, within a particular weight range – and the lives of many people are endangered by a system that all too often does not account for medical variation from this faulty and limited standard. Thinking about the contemporary problems and practices of gynaecological medicine does not draw attention away from, but rather enriches study of, the gynaecological concerns of early medieval women in England. Systemic treatment of these bodies, both then and now, bears out the markers of a patriarchal system that has endangered, and continues to endanger, the lives of women and people giving birth.

This shortsightedness was true, too, in early medieval England. The medical tradition demonstrates little concern for women's illness, particularly for childbirth, probably one of the leading causes of death in women aged between fifteen and forty-five. Despite the imminent danger presented by childbirth, the most common subject of remedies in relation to women's bodies is menstruation. Menstruation is enormously important; it is indicative of the health of a woman, of her status with regard to conception and childbearing, and of her safety after birth. Menstruation is of concern both in its presence and in its absence, as well as in its quality and duration. The textual focus on menstruation instead of childbirth reveals a concern with the reproductive viability of women, leaving the actual processes of childbirth up to (textually absent) midwives. The primary medical concern with women's bodies is about controlling and harnessing menstruation in service of fertility.

Women must be able to produce children as part of the social contract; indeed, ensuring regular menses is a basic component of treatment for infertility. And yet, embedded in the language of 'provoking flow' is a notion of control over reproductive potential; such remedies *could* be used to hamper as well as to promote fertility. These medical texts, written and read by men, offer knowledge to promote fertility and attempt to regulate and dominate women's bodies and what they produce. But even as such learned texts silence the voices of women by overwriting actual practice and bodies with textual ones, they cannot fully efface the desires of women, which are not always consistent with the desires of the patriarchal systems they inhabit. Through their attempts to promote and harness women's fertility by controlling menstruation, the medical texts also, paradoxically, indicate the potential for women to regulate their own menses and fertility according to their own desires.

In thinking about the kinds of erasure and effacement of women through the mechanisms of masculine supremacy and universality, I reconstitute the generalised category of 'reproductive medicine' through a feminist praxis of linguistic interrogation and careful close reading. Doing so reveals a tradition that does in fact seek to treat the birthing bodies of women, although the language for these practices has been obscured in a number of ways, from its inception, to its early manuscript studies and translations, to the work of contemporary scholars and our tools. This project works to understand the experiences, as much as is possible, of ordinary early medieval women, but also to see the reflections of these practices in the contemporary treatment (and effacement) of women's reproductive maladies.

Women's maladies, women's agency, women's erasure

This book traces the processes of an early medieval woman's reproductive cycle, beginning with menstruation and ending with cleansing. The perspective of these texts is necessarily male – the voice of practitioner, expert, author – but the subject is the body of a woman who seeks help. While the women in these remedies do not exactly speak, neither are they silent. They ask, how can I be healed? They say, here are my symptoms. They intone the incantations and prayers provided to them by the experts. They leave behind objects that hint at their individual stories, and they leave behind their bodies as texts to be read and understood with both curiosity and empathy. They do not occupy the position of expert in the authorial voices of these texts, but there is no text without them. Similarly, the manuscripts packed full of remedies make little space for these few remedies directed at the bodies of women, and yet even their paucity and absence tell a story. Perhaps it is a story of the helping women whose work and knowledge do not matter to the social order at large, or perhaps it is a story of women for whom there is little help at all. Perhaps, however, it is a story about the networks of women who travel, as Sayer suggests, to live, give birth and die in communities filled with other women like them, ciphers in the literary tradition, but present in the archaeological, and even perhaps the medical, ones.[59]

This book uses medical texts written and deployed by patriarchal authorities in order to think about the ways such texts offer a vision of women as objects but also agents determining the patterns of their lives through the medical help they required. Chapter 1 discusses women as diagnostic subjects via the language around menstruation and the kinds of remedies and ingredients used to treat and address menstrual irregularities. The chapter calls into question the work of nineteenth-century translators and dictionaries that work to obscure menstrual remedies and the desired functions of these treatments. Chapter 2 turns away from close attention to language for maladies in order to think about the nature of time and agency relative to remedies and prognostics for fertility and pregnancy, wherein male practitioners attempt to enact controls over women's bodies, but also establish frameworks that hold women accountable for problems with fertility and undesirable pregnancy outcomes.

Chapter 3 returns to a close examination of the language of childbirth, working to make distinct the terms *cennan*, *geeacnian*, *geberan*, and *gefedan*, all of which translators over time have rendered to mean 'giving birth', without thoughtful consideration of the content or relationships between these terms and their manuscript contexts. This chapter pulls together the threads of Chapters 1 and 2, working to develop the idea of a woman as an agent who has authority in her own process of birth, and of grieving births that do not come to fruition. Finally, Chapter 4 interweaves threads from all the previous chapters, thinking through problems of agency and authority manifested in the deployment and understanding of timelines for pregnancy and pregnancy loss in the early medieval period. It continues the close attention to language as it seeks to distinguish between ideas of purging (*afeormian*) and cleansing (*clænsian*), which have previously been conflated in a general response that reflects the abjection of women's bodies. Ultimately, these chapters work together to paint a picture of an early medieval woman whose access to information about her own medical and reproductive identity is delimited in specific ways by figures in positions of authority, an effacement of her autonomy that is accreted over time through acts of occlusive and apathetic translation and glossing. And yet, the nature of the woman's reproductive cycles, the timing of which presses against the expectations and approval of authorities, suggests that she was able to exert control over her own reproductive destiny and identity through the kinds of remedies present in the medical tradition.

Notes

1 Thomas Oswald Cockayne, *Leechdoms, wortcunning, and starcraft of early England. Being a collection of documents, for the most part never before printed, illustrating the history of science in this country before the Norman Conquest*, 3 vols (London: Longman, Green, Longman, Roberts and Green, 1864–66), Vol. II, p. 306.
2 Ibid., Vol. II, p. 309.
3 Anne Van Arsdall, *Medieval Herbal Remedies: The Old English Herbarium and Anglo-Saxon Medicine* (London: Routledge, 2022), p. 119.
4 *Bald's Leechbook* appears with *Leechbook III* in the tenth-century MS Royal 12.D.xvii, and features 1,129 remedies. My eternal gratitude goes to Christine Voth for her expertise on this manuscript and her generosity in sharing her knowledge and insights about its many strangenesses. Please see Voth's excellent scholarship both in her forthcoming edition (Debby Banham and Christine Voth (eds and trans), *Old English Medicine in British Library, Royal D. xvii*, Vol. II of *Anglo-Saxon Medical Texts*, Dumbarton Oaks Medieval Library (Cambridge, MA: Harvard University Press, forthcoming)), and her PhD thesis ('An Analysis of the Tenth-Century Anglo-Saxon Manuscript London, British Library, Royal 12.D.xvii' (University of Cambridge, 2015)). The total count of remedies was shared in personal correspondence (6 October 2021), wherein she delineates the breakdown of remedies as 580 from Book I, 390 surviving remedies from Book II (she notes 'I do include the remedies copied from Book Two into another manuscript (Chapter 59)', and 169 in Book III (where she notes that the last chapters are missing). This count therefore relays existing remedies, and not remedies that appear only in the table of contents, without other existing versions.
5 Voth, 'Analysis', p. 147.
6 Voth notes consistent variations between the numbers as listed in the table of contents and those that exist in the manuscript. She suggests that this may be a way of addressing duplicates, or simple miscounting (ibid., p. 139). She notes that the remedies do not seem to be missing as the result of damage.
7 Despite assumptions that it was primarily religious men who were literate at the time, scholars including Susanmarie Harrington argue that religious women and some of the laity also participated in literate culture as both readers and writers. See Susanmarie Harrington, 'Women, Literacy, and Intellectual Culture in Anglo-Saxon England', PhD thesis (University of Michigan, 1990).

8 The Ancientbiotics project is a 'cross-disciplinary team of medievalists and scientists from different disciplines who are interested in the remedies from historical and traditional medicine … Medicine in the Middle Ages could take many forms and medical remedies are only a part of it. Our project considers medieval pharmacology and one of our aims is to investigate whether any of the remedies may be adapted to help to find new solutions for modern problems, such as a rise in antimicrobial resistance'; https://ancientbiotics.co.uk/ (accessed 14 June 2023).
9 Voth, 'Analysis', p. 17. See especially the work of Maria D'Aronco (John Niles and Maria D'Aronco (eds and trans), *Anglo-Saxon Medical Texts*, Vol. I, *The Old English Herbal, Lacnunga, and Other Texts*, Dumbarton Oaks Medieval Library (Cambridge, MA: Harvard University Press, 2023)); Anne Van Arsdall (*Medieval Herbal Remedies*); Debby Banham (with Christine Voth, *Old English Medicine*); Audrey Meaney (*Anglo-Saxon Amulets and Curing Stones* (Oxford: British Archaeological Reports, 1981)); Karen Jolly (*Popular Religion in Late Saxon England: Elf Charms in Context* (Charlotte: University of North Carolina Press, 1996)); Emily Kesling (*Medical Texts in Anglo-Saxon Literary Culture* (Cambridge: D. S. Brewer, 2020)); and Lori Ann Garner (*Hybrid Healing: Old English Remedies and Medical Texts* (Manchester: Manchester University Press, 2022)).
10 David Wootton, *Bad Medicine: Doctors Doing Harm since Hippocrates* (Oxford: Oxford University Press, 2007), p. 17; Peregrine Horden, 'What's Wrong with Early Medieval Medicine?', *Social History of Medicine*, 24.1 (2009), 5–25 (p. 20).
11 Horden, 'What's Wrong?', p. 20.
12 Erin Sweany, 'Unsettling Comparisons: Ethical Considerations of Comparative Approaches to the Old English Medical Corpus', *English Language Notes*, 58.2 (October 2020), 83–100 (p. 86).
13 I have used a range of editions in the preparation of this book. The texts of *OEH*, *OEM* and *Lacnunga* are from Niles and D'Aronco, *Anglo-Saxon Medical Texts*, Vol. I. They offer slightly different titles for these texts (the *Old English Herbal* and *Old English Remedies from Animals*, respectively), but I retain versions of the titles that have appeared generally in previous scholarship. At the time of writing, the second of the Dumbarton Oaks editions of the texts has not yet been published (*Old English Medicine in British Library, Royal D. xvii, Anglo-Saxon Medical Texts*, Vol. II, Dumbarton Oaks Medieval Library (Cambridge, MA: Harvard University Press, forthcoming)), although the editors have shared generously their expertise and

early drafts of their editions of *LBIII* and *Bald*. Citations from these sources come from Cockayne, *Leechdoms*. I have looked to editions and translations, including Hubert Jan de Vriend (ed.), *The Old English Herbarium and Medicina de Quadrupedibus*, Early English Text Society (Oxford: Oxford University Press, 1984); Van Arsdall, *Medieval Herbal Remedies*; and Edward Thomas Pettit (ed. and trans.), *Anglo-Saxon Remedies, Charms, and Prayers from the British Library MS Harley 585: The Lacnunga*, 2 vols (Lewiston: Edwin Mellen Press, 2001). I regularly use Cockayne as a reference, although Cockayne is often a problematic editor, cutting or refusing to translate certain remedies that he finds objectionable. I discuss this problem at greater length in the following chapters.

14 London, British Library (BL), MS Cotton Vitellius CIII; Oxford, Bodleian Library, MS Hatton 76; and BL, MS Harley 6358B, the last of which, as Kesling notes, dates at the latest from the twelfth century, although the earlier manuscripts place the composition of the collection in the late tenth century (Kesling, *Medical Texts*, p. 6 n. 10).

15 Ibid., p. 5.

16 In general, Kesling's work offers an important corrective to many of the early studies on medicine that identify these Old English sources as primitive and superstitious, often ignoring their strong connections to the larger medieval medical context. Important early works that have required this sort of corrective response include J. H. G. Grattan, *Anglo-Saxon Magic and Medicine* (Oxford: Oxford University Press, 1952); M. L. Cameron, *Anglo-Saxon Medicine* (Cambridge: Cambridge University Press, 1993); and Wilfrid Bonser, who in 1963 critiqued the deplorable state of early medieval English concern with obstetrics, saying 'the writings of Greek and Latin authors on obstetrics had not penetrated to this island, and … knowledge of the subject was at its lowest ebb', in *The Medical Background of Anglo-Saxon England* (London: Publications of the Wellcome Historical Library, 1963), p. 264.

17 Van Arsdall, *Medieval Herbal Remedies*, p. 71.

18 Van Arsdall claims that multiple translations of the *OEH* exist in order to 'make it more accessible to Anglo-Saxon speakers who consulted it; it was not viewed as some kind of esoteric treatise that was beyond the reach of practitioners … on the contrary, it was an essential text' (ibid., p. 75). Furthermore, she emphasises that 'the monasteries and monks of Anglo-Saxon England were part of this European-wide system of healing, where apprenticeship, word-of-mouth information, tradition, and texts all contributed to the healer's art' (p. 82).

19 Kesling, *Medical Texts*, p. 22. I endeavour to avoid this phrase wherever possible in this book because of its associations with a long tradition of white supremacy. I retain it inside existing quotations and in the titles of sources. I am grateful to the work of scholars including Mary Rambaran-Olm and Adam Miyashiro for their work in laying bare the cultural assumptions embedded in this language. See Mary Rambaran-Olm, 'Anglo-Saxon Studies [Early English Studies], Academia and White Supremacy', *Medium* (27 June 2018), https://mrambaranolm.medium.com/anglo-saxon-studies-academia-and-white-supremacy-17c87b360bf3 (accessed 25 October 2021); Mary Rambaran-Olm, 'History Bites: Resources on the Problematic Term "Anglo-Saxon", Part 1', *Medium* (7 September 2020), https://mrambaranolm.medium.com/history-bites-resources-on-the-problematic-term-anglo-saxon-part-1–9320b6a09eb7 Mary (accessed 25 April 2022); Mary Rambaran-Olm, 'Misnaming the Medieval: Rejecting "Anglo-Saxon" Studies', *History Workshop* (4 November 2019), www.historyworkshop.org.uk/misnaming-the-medieval-rejecting-anglo-saxon-studies/ (accessed 25 October 2021); Mary Rambaran-Olm, with Erik Wade, 'The Many Myths of the Term "Anglo-Saxon"', *Smithsonian Magazine* (14 July 2021), www.smithsonianmag.com/history/many-myths-term-anglo-saxon-180978169/ (accessed 25 October 2021); and Adam Miyashiro, 'Decolonizing Anglo-Saxon Studies: A Response to ISAS in Honolulu', *In the Middle* (29 July 2017), www.inthemedievalmiddle.com/2017/07/decolonizing-anglo-saxon-studies.html (accessed 25 October 2021). See also Mary Rambaran-Olm's list of resources on the term in 'History Bites: Resources on the Problematic Term "Anglo-Saxon", Part 3', *Medium* (7 September 2020), https://mrambaranolm.medium.com/history-bites-resources-on-the-problematic-term-anglo-saxon-part-3-2f38919569f0 (accessed 25 October 2021).
20 Peregrine Horden further suggests the inadequacy of the textual tradition relative to actual practice, adding that 'most techniques were transmitted orally and through clinical experience. The role of texts was limited and oblique, even in the most literate settings'; Horden, 'What's Wrong?', p. 18.
21 Cameron, *Anglo-Saxon Medicine*, p. 19.
22 Stanley Rubin's 1970 article assumes without qualification a male-only practitioner, discussing medical treatment in monastic and non-monastic houses, and referring only once to women, in order to discuss the advice for dietary restrictions for pregnant women; Stanley Rubin, 'The Medical Practitioner in Anglo-Saxon England', *Journal of the Royal College of General Practitioners*, 20.97 (1970),

63–71. In 'Women and "Women's Medicine", Early Medieval England: From Text to Practice', in R. Trilling, R. Norris and R. Stephenson (eds), *Feminist Approaches to Anglo-Saxon Studies* (Amsterdam: Amsterdam University Press, 2023), pp. 279–316, Christine Voth examines the potential female ownership of the manuscript containing the Royal Prayer Book, citing the work of both Michelle Brown and Jennifer Morrish, both of whom suggest that a female physician may have owned this manuscript. See also Roberta Gilchrist's *Sacred Heritage: Monastic Archeology, Identities, Beliefs* (Cambridge: Cambridge University Press, 2020), which expands the conversation about medieval medicine to include preventative care. Voth claims that material sources via archaeology 'provide new perspectives on the broader empirical tradition delivered by a diverse range of practitioners – physicians (often monks and priests), surgeons, bone-setters, apothecaries, herbalists, lay-sisters and midwives', in 'Women and "Women's Medicine"', p. 78.
23 Fiona Harris Stoertz, 'Suffering and Survival in Medieval English Childbirth', in Cathy Jorgensen Itnyre (ed.), *Medieval Family Roles* (Hoboken, NJ: Garland Press, 1996), pp. 101–20 (p. 103).
24 I discuss this term and its intricacies in greater detail in Chapter 1.
25 Cameron, *Anglo-Saxon Medicine*, p. 22.
26 Monica Green, 'Gendering the History of Women's Healthcare', *Gender & History*, 20.3 (2008), 487–518 (p. 490).
27 Ibid., p. 496.
28 Emily Kesling, 'The Old English Medical Collections in the Literary Context', PhD thesis (Oxford University, 2016), p. 200. Lori Ann Garner, in her 2023 conference presentation at Kalamazoo, noted the variations among *OEH* manuscripts, offering potential explanations for why certain remedies were excluded from some manuscripts. In her monograph, she examines the distinctions between the *Herbarium* as it appears in Cotton Vitellius C.iii and in the later manuscript, Harley 6258B, noting that deletions of certain treatments indicate 'another clear shift away from a model of plant agency' (*Hybrid Healing*, p. 187).
29 Antoinette diPaolo Healey, with John Price Wilkin and Xin Xiang (eds), *Dictionary of Old English Web Corpus* (Toronto: Dictionary of Old English Project, 2009).
30 These non-gynaecological remedies do not always specify that they are for women, although some do. They total fewer than fifteen remedies. Those for breast pain are *OEH* 5.5, 19.3, 116.1, 117.2, 149.1 and 173.3; those for sexual pleasure include *OEM* 3.13, 3.14, 4.10, 6.11, 9.08, 10.13 and 12.14. Thanks to Christine Voth for identifying and

classifying these remedies. The prognostics, discussed in Chapter 3, also include relevant medical-adjacent material, for instance charting the development of a foetus in the womb, and signs of pregnancy, but these texts are distinct from remedies.

31 R. A. Buck suggests a male author for the leechbooks: 'There are a number of linguistic clues throughout the [Anglo-Saxon] Leechbooks that identify men, rather than women, as the writers and compilers of the medical treatises'; 'Woman's Milk in Anglo-Saxon and Later Medieval Medical Texts', *Neophilologus*, 96.3 (2012), 467–85 (p. 469).

32 By exceptional, I mean that the women who appear in Old English literature tend to be extremely high-status figures: powerful abbesses, biblical heroines, queens and the Virgin Mary. It is difficult to find ordinary women in this literary tradition.

33 Clare Lees and Gillian Overing, *Double Agents: Women and Clerical Culture in Anglo-Saxon England* (Philadelphia: University of Pennsylvania Press, 2001).

34 Gale R. Owen-Crocker, 'Anglo-Saxon Women, Woman, and Womanhood', in Helene Scheck and Christine E. Kozikowski (eds), *New Readings on Women and Early Medieval English Literature and Culture: Cross-Disciplinary Studies in Honour of Helen Damico* (Amsterdam: Amsterdam University Press, 2019), pp. 23–41 (pp. 32–3).

35 Duncan Sayer and Sam D. Dickinson, 'Reconsidering Obstetric Death and Female Fertility in Anglo-Saxon England', *World Archaeology*, 45.2 (2013), 285–97 (p. 291).

36 Sally Crawford, *Childhood in Anglo-Saxon England* (Stroud: Sutton, 1999), p. 63.

37 Sayer and Dickinson, 'Reconsidering Obstetric Death', p. 286.

38 Caroline R. Batten, '"Lazarus, Come Forth": Pregnancy and Childbirth in the Life Course of Early Medieval English Women', in Thijs Porck and Harriet Soper (eds), *Early Medieval English Life Courses: Cultural-Historical Perspectives* (Leiden: Brill, 2022), pp. 140–58 (p. 147).

39 Sayer and Dickinson, 'Reconsidering Obstetric Death', p. 286.

40 Ibid., p. 291.

41 Owen-Crocker, 'Anglo-Saxon Women', p. 34.

42 Sayer and Dickinson, 'Reconsidering Obstetric Death', p. 290.

43 Ibid., p. 293.

44 According to *DOE Web Corpus*, *wamb* occurs 245 times, 101 of these in the medical texts, none of which refer to women's wombs explicitly. A close study of these occurrences would be valuable.

45 Joseph Bosworth, 'INNOÞ', in *An Anglo-Saxon Dictionary Online*, ed. Thomas Northcote Toller, Christ Sean, and Ondřej Tichy (Prague: Faculty of Arts, Charles University, 2014), https://bosworthtoller.com/20658 (accessed 23 December 2023) (hereafter Bosworth–Toller).

46 Jane Roberts, Christian Kay and Lynne Grundy, 'penis', in *A Thesaurus of Old English* (Leiden: Brill, 2000), https://oldenglishthesaurus.arts.gla.ac.uk/ (accessed 9 January 2018). According to Bosworth–Toller, *lim* means 'a limb, joint, member of a body, branch of a tree' (according to the *DOE Web Corpus*, 88 discrete occurrences, many of which may not refer to the penis); *pintel* means 'virilitas, membrum virile' (only one occurrence, as a gloss); *sceamlim* means 'the private member' (also only one occurrence as a gloss); *teors* again means 'membrum virile'; and *wæpen*, after 'weapon' as its first meaning, lists 'membrum virile' as its second (twenty-six occurrences, most of which do not refer to the penis). It is notable, if not surprising, that these nineteenth-century research tools refuse to use the word 'penis', and resort to Latin.

47 In a search of the *DOE Web Corpus*, *matrix* occurs seven times, only in glosses. Terms that appear as glosses for *matrix* include *cildhama* (eight occurrences, all as glosses); *cennincge* (four occurrences; two occur in verb form and refer to birth; the other occurrences are glosses, one for birth and one for *matrix*); *eacnuncge* (in a single gloss); *quiða* (three occurrences as glosses); and *wifmannas innoþ* (in a single gloss).

48 Bosworth–Toller, 'ge-cynd-lim', https://bosworthtoller.com/14003. Not all of these occurrences refer to women's bodies, and two occur in *OEM*, in one case referring to the body part of a deer, the other to a swollen body part. In both cases it is unclear if the referent is a penis or a uterus, or another perceived generative organ.

49 On Galenic medicine and the one-sex model, see Thomas Laqueur, *Making Sex: Body and Gender from the Greeks to Freud* (Cambridge: Harvard University Press, 1990). We might see this as a reflection of the generalisation of all bodies, the flattening out of gender into a single category. The trouble, of course, is that that single category is male. Medieval people, like contemporary ones, did not experience gender as this simple male/female binary, but rather existed in the world in a range of ways, and in bodies that may or may not have fitted neatly into binaries or social and even medical expectations. See also Blake Gutt, who, with Alicia Spencer-Hall, argues '"Transgender" is not just an identity, or a form of embodiment, but a way of disrupting normative and essentializing

frameworks', and further that 'Medieval and modern conception of gender – what it is, how it is produced, why it matters – differ. Yet in both periods, there are gender norms, and transgressions thereof.' Blake Gutt and Alicia Spencer-Hall, 'Introduction', in Blake Gutt and Alicia Spencer-Hall (eds), *Trans and Genderqueer Subjects in Medieval Hagiography* (Amsterdam: Amsterdam University Press, 2021), pp. 11–40 (pp. 13–14). See also Robert Mills, *Seeing Sodomy in the Middle Ages* (Chicago: University of Chicago Press, 2015).
50 Leah DeVun, *The Shape of Sex: Nonbinary Gender from Genesis to the Renaissance* (New York: Columbia University Press, 2021), p. 115.
51 See Rambaran-Olm, 'History Bites, Part 1'. Rambaran-Olm serves as one of the many voices of critique for the scholarly field and its name; she argues that 'the term "Anglo-Saxon" itself is anachronistic as it carries the baggage of 19th-century racial hierarchies'. In this book, I use this term only when inside direct quotations or titled works.
52 Thanks to Adam Miyashiro for contextualising the colonial history of the Early English Text Society in his talk 'Race, White Supremacy, and the Middle Ages', International Congress on Medieval Studies, Western Michigan University, 13 May 2018. See also Adam Miyashiro, '"Our Deeper Past": Race, Settler Colonialism, and Medieval Heritage Politics', *Literature Compass*, 16 (2019), 1–11, where he argues that 'The version of the "Saxon myth" that emerged in North America in the 18th and 19th centuries was shaped by various political and academic forces that changed significantly the contours of how the term "Anglo-Saxon" became racialized' (p. 5), and further that British histories promoting a 'romantic interpretation of Anglo-Saxon law and Tacitus' *Germania*' were informed by law but also by philology (p. 6). We must use these tools with awareness, and replace them when they no longer serve us. The new Dumbarton Oaks series on medical texts is a prime example of this much-needed action. So too will the *DOE*'s continuing work promote these important changes.
53 CDC Newsroom, 'Racial and Ethnic Disparities Continue in Pregnancy-Related Death' (6 September 2019), www.cdc.gov/media/releases/2019/p0905-racial-ethnic-disparities-pregnancy-deaths.html (accessed 27 June 2023).
54 'Black Women and Reproductive Health', *In Our Own Voice: National Black Women's Reproductive Justice Agenda*, http://blackrj.org/wp-content/uploads/2015/10/BlackWomen-andReproductiveHealthFS.pdf (accessed 27 June 2023). See also *Reimagining Policy: In Pursuit*

of *Black Reproductive Justice*, 2023 Black Reproductive Justice Policy Agenda, https://blackrj.org/blackrjpolicyagenda/ (accessed 27 June 2023).
55 Deirdre Cooper Owens, 'Listening to Black Women Saves Black Lives', *Lancet*, 397.10276 (27 February 2021), 788–9 (p. 789).
56 Imogen Learmonth, 'The Gender Health Gap: Why Women's Bodies Shouldn't Be a Medical Mystery', Thred media (September 2020), https://thred.com/change/the-gender-health-gap-why-womens-bodies-shouldnt-be-a-medical-mystery/ (accessed 3 November 2021). For thorough treatment of the data around this issue, see Caroline Criado Perez, *Invisible Women: Data Bias in a World Designed for Men* (New York: Abrams Press, 2019). See also Lea Merone, Komla Tsey, Darren Russell and Cate Nagle, 'Sex Inequalities in Medical Research: A Systematic Scoping Review of the Literature', *Women's Health Reports*, 3.1 (2022): 49–59. They conclude that 'the gender gap and misogynistic studies, which serve little to improve women's health, remain present in the contemporary literature' (p. 59). Many studies demonstrate discrepancies in research and treatment, including Jecca R. Steinbert, Brandon E. Turner, Brannon T. Weeks et al., 'Analysis of Female Enrollment and Participant Sex by Burden of Disease in US Clinical Trials between 2000 and 2020', *JAMA Network Open*, 4.6 (2021), DOI: 10.1001/jamanetworkopen.2021.13749; and Brad N. Greenwood, Seth Carnahan, and Laura Huang, 'Patient–Physician Gender Concordance and Increased Mortality among Female Heart Attack Patients', *Proceedings of the National Academy of Sciences*, 115.34 (6 August 2018), 8569–74, DOI: 10.1073/pnas.1800097115.
57 Learmonth, 'The Gender Health Gap'.
58 Nicola Slawson, '"Women Have Been Woefully Neglected": Does Medical Science Have a Gender Problem?', *Guardian* (18 December 2019), www.theguardian.com/education/2019/dec/18/women-have-been-woefully-neglected-does-medical-science-have-a-gender-problem (accessed 3 November 2021). Furthermore, Lisa Mosconi cites research by Caroline Criado Perez, wherein 'they studied Viagra, and they found that with women, it completely eliminated period cramps for four hours at a time with no side effects. And the doctor that discovered this went back to the NIH [National Institutes of Health], twice, and said, "We need further studies on this. This is the holy grail for women", and they said, "Well, dysmenorrhea is not a real issue." So we now know everything we need to know about penises and how they get hard, and how Viagra can make them harder, but nothing about how Viagra could be helping the other 50% of the population, enormously.' Lisa Mosconi, 'Exploring

the Link between Menopause and Alzheimer's', *Medium* (30 May 2019), https://medium.com/neurotrack/menopause-and-alzheimers-1c455f29fe16 (accessed 3 November 2021).

59 Duncan Sayer, '"Sons of Athelings Given to the Earth": Infant Mortality within Anglo-Saxon Mortuary Geography', *Medieval Archaeology*, 58.1 (2014), 78–103 (p. 97).

1

The diagnostic body and the matter of menstruation in the remedies and penitentials

Famously, NASA engineers preparing to send Sally Ride into space believed that she might need 100 tampons for her week-long sojourn.[1] Social media posts about men's wild misunderstandings about menstruation abound, more than forty years later, including gems like a teacher who told a young woman to 'hold it' until class was over, and a man who believes that women experience only nine periods per year and require a maximum of seven tampons per menstrual cycle, who used this logic to scold women for objecting to taxation for menstrual products. In the United States of America, tampons and menstrual products are not included in tax-exempt status, like other medical necessities, although several states are working to eliminate the tampon tax. Notably, the state in which I live, Wisconsin, is not one of them. The financial costs of menstruation are one part of a more complex social milieu that demonises people for living in bodies that menstruate. In 2019, the United Nations rights experts identified menstrual autonomy as a human right, calling for an end to 'the taboo around menstrual health for women and girls that persists in many parts of the world'.[2] The United Nations Population Fund notes that 'over the lifetime of a person who menstruates, they could easily spend three to eight years menstruating, during which they might face menstrual-related exclusion, neglect, or discrimination'.[3] The first prong of a four-prong approach to achieving global menstrual health begins with changing structural attitudes to menstruation, in part by 'including men and boys, along with those who menstruate, towards reducing menstrual stigma, which is often a product of patriarchal norms'.[4]

Cultural stigmas have been attached to menstruation for millennia. The Judeo-Christian tradition figures menstruation as a woman's curse, a specifically feminine punishment for the sins of Eve. In medieval penitential culture, menstruation is treated as a kind of pollution, requiring shame, the barring of entry to the church and abstention from sex. Exclusive to the bodies of women, it is understood in the majority of Old English texts as a malady, a disease, a punishment and an unnamable process. Old English does not have a single, unified way of naming or understanding menstruation. Despite the lack of coherent vocabulary and the religious taboos around it, the regulation of menstruation is the most prominent concern of the Old English medical texts for the bodies of women. This category accounts for the largest proportion of women's remedies, and includes treatments for women who wish to start a reluctant or absent period, or to stop an excessive one.

In a literal way, this chapter is concerned with the nature of presence and absence in the same sense as medieval women and practitioners were; it is concerned with what to do when a menstrual period is present – in some cases, far too present – but also with what to do when a period is absent, and all the attendant concerns over causes and consequences of the absence of menstruation. The treatments in the medical texts specific to menstruation, either provoking or preventing it, demonstrate the complex interplay of agency between the person asking for help, the authority who offers it, and the social circumstances that inform these critical events in a woman's life. By thinking carefully about the language used to depict women's bodies, organs, processes and problems, we can more fully understand the social perception of the bodies of ordinary early English women. Further, by considering the implications of authority and expert (read: male) diagnosis and control over women's maladies by the regulation of their menstruation, we can think about the complex dynamics that exist between the laity and the clergy, but also between women and the many editors, translators and glossators of texts who have inserted their own gendered anxieties and social taboos into the perpetuation of the text. The covering over of menstruation, often by means of burying in Latin or other euphemistic language, exists in a long tradition of textual mediation, fixed as it is in each historical moment. Each act of mediation perpetuates and re-engineers a set of taboos regarding menstruation and the bodies of women that has continuously endangered the lives of women.

The early sections of this chapter consider the relationships between Old English penitential and medical texts, first arguing that both genres establish what I term the diagnostic body. Both genres operate within a call-and-response structure, one that establishes the relationship between a seeker of help and a purveyor of relief via extra special (textual) expertise. While this dynamic might seem to prop up the authority of the expert (the confessor or the physician), in fact it also establishes the self-recognition and agency that accompany self-declaration and the request for help. As two of the only genres that depict menstruating bodies, penitentials and medical texts are critical to understanding the perception of menstruation, but they use distinct vocabulary in order to describe it. While penitential texts emphasise taboos regarding menstruation, the taboos that appear in the medical texts often arrive courtesy of later translators as much as, or perhaps more than, original practitioners and authors. The medical texts, once we have separated out the anxieties of nineteenth-century translators and glossators, provide a refreshingly overt discussion of the needs of women's bodies and the importance of regular, healthy menstruation.

However pleasingly frank the discussion of menstruation in the medical texts, they do not offer a comprehensive or accurate understanding of menstruation that the treatments of menstrual irregularities require. The remedies for menstruation fall into two general categories – those for stopping flow and those for provoking it – which I treat in separate sections. The remedies that seek to stop excessive flow treat only the symptom and rarely the cause of a flow that will not cease. However, in those remedies for provoking flow, I argue for subtle distinctions wherein underlying causes are far more likely to be addressed than in the case of remedies for stopping flow. While ensuring healthy menstruation is a fundamental element of fertility, I suggest that those remedies for provoking flow walk a fine line between ensuring the continuation of the patriarchal structure by fulfilling the social contract to produce children, and offering women a potential agency over their own reproductive identities.

The diagnostic body in the penitentials and medical remedies

Remedies, by their very nature, set up the dynamic of asking and answering. In suggesting that, for example, yarrow is good for snakebite, the text sets up an implicit question and an asker: a person who, in this instance, quite desperately, needs an answer to 'what can I do for a snakebite?'.[5] In the asking of the question, the body of the asker is conjured forth, bitten and in need of care. It is a body in crisis, and so is both a kind of universal, but also a specific; *this* body needs a cure for snakebite, but also *enough bodies* require this cure for a category to exist. The remedies anticipate the question 'what can I do for *my* toothache?', with the answer 'If a person has a toothache …'. In this way, the remedies function very much like the penitentials. Przemysław Tyszka clarifies that:

> Men and women in penitentials (as in other historical sources) were not presented as abstract personifications of masculinity or femininity. They appeared there as representatives of specific categories – the clergy (divided into subgroups), laymen, husbands, wives, virgins, widows, boys, bachelors etc. In classifying sinners the authors of the penitentials drew attention to their functions and positions within the cult community, their marital status and age.[6]

The penitentials respond to the question 'what should I do to be absolved for this action?' and thereby call forth the body that has performed such an action. They suggest that individual sinners can be absolved, but also that individual sinners occupy a category that is shared by other such sinners. This rhetorical communal singularity – a need that is at once individual and also shared – is embraced by both penitential and medical texts, and is fundamental to their structure.

The trouble with the penitentials, as with the remedies, lies in our inability to detect how frequently they were used and if they truly represent the kinds of behaviours being enacted by early medieval people. Erik Wade notes that many scholars 'have been reluctant to view the penitentials as reliable historical evidence, particularly for sexual behaviour, doubting how much effect they had on everyday life and even suggesting that they were largely unused', citing, as an example, Christine Fell's decision to avoid the penitentials as evidence.[7] But he also notes Pierre Payer's critique of this dismissal, wherein he suggests that scholars are content to use the penitentials to understand other types of sin, while casting doubt only on sexual sins. Wade rejects these critiques of the penitentials as removed from the real and lived experiences of early medieval people through his examination of the anonymous woman who seeks the advice of Theodore regarding her current marriage (which took place after an earlier vow of celibacy). He states:

> Her 'deviation' is not sensationalized. Rather, her petition and Theodore's gentle judgment are evidence of everyday piety and illustrate that marriage and sexuality were indeed pressing concerns for the laity. Some secular women apparently spent much time and energy considering the theological significance of their everyday actions as well as appropriate Christian behaviour in their marriages. The [*Pœnitentiale Theodori*] was a direct response to these concerns, which helps to account for its popularity, diffuse manuscript transmission, and subsequent influence.[8]

In one tidy passage, Wade defends the use of the penitentials to understand the real penitential desires of the laity, and of women specifically, arguing that the penitentials ultimately construct women as 'theological and legal subjects for the first time', and not merely as the property of men.[9] Similarly, this structuring of need specific to women in the remedies provides a kind of access to the bodies of women that exists nowhere else in the corpus of Old English writing.

If the penitentials bring forth the voices of women participating in conversations and negotiations about spiritual matters, so too do the remedies present us with people asking for help, implicitly, from religious and textual authorities – from those who act as experts and conveyers of knowledge. In this sense, both the medical texts and the penitentials present us with what I term the diagnostic body. Both genres imagine a real body in need of healing, be it spiritual or medical, whether or not the writing of such texts grew from interaction with real bodies or not. In this way, it does not matter that we do not know how 'useful' the remedies might have been, or if real people got up to all the activities, sexual and otherwise, that we find in the penitentials. Both sets of texts attempt to imagine real bodies with real questions, and in so doing they give us access to the real bodies of actual people. These are not literary figures, set up as ideals, evacuated from their bodily natures. These are not good queens or ambitious thanes or heroic pagans. These are ordinary bodies, exceptional only in that they stand in for whole categories of suffering bodies or spirits.

Menstrual terminology in medical and penitential texts

In a textual tradition that rarely features women at all, menstruation specifically allows women to appear in both the medical texts and penitentials, rather than being subsumed under the general category of man/person. Despite the fact that half of the adult population of early medieval England had experienced menstruation, the language for this function appears, for the most part, in only these two genres, with rare appearances in other religious texts (e.g. Bede's report of Augustine's correspondence with Pope Gregory; the story of Veronica). That such a mundane occurrence appears so rarely demonstrates the taboos with which it is associated, as well as the narrow worldview of authors. In a surprising way, however, menstruation invites women's bodies and the bodies of those who menstruate into a literary tradition that frequently excludes them. That is, because menstruation is specific to certain kinds of bodies, and because there are medical treatments for menstruation, those bodies appear in texts not *in spite of* but *because of* their taboo bodily function.[10] If we read generously, including glosses and making space for uncertain usages, menstruation is discussed fewer than sixty times in the entire corpus of Old English writing; this number includes the entirety of medical, legal, penitential, biblical and literary occurrences. And yet, of women's health concerns, menstruation receives the greatest percentage of remedies.

The language for menstruation in Old English is varied, and depends on genre. Much of the language used to describe menstruation applies also to bloodflow more generally, as is the case with terms like *blodryne* ('blood-running') and *flewsan* (flow). Alternatively, language for menstruation often refers to its cyclical timing and 'monthliness', as with *monoðlican* ('monthlies'), *monaðgecynd* ('of monthly nature'), *monaðadle* ('monthly illness') and, surprisingly rarely, *monaðblod* ('monthly blood'). Although there is some overlap between penitential and medical language for menstruation (as with *blodryne* and *flewsan*), penitential texts favour language that pathologises menstruation (*monaðadle*), whereas medical ones employ less value-laden language. In short, the penitentials enforce menstrual taboos;

medical texts treat menstrual concerns without condemnation or judgement, and the language each chooses reflects this distinction. Indeed, later translators are the most frequent culprits in forwarding taboo notions in medical texts, as they struggle with how to convey menstruation politely to their own (squeamish) audiences.

Not all of this language for menstruation functions synonymously; terms like *blodryne* seem to refer to a specific malady and not to general menstruation. The emphatic phrase *blodryne*, translated in Bosworth–Toller as 'blood-coursing', and in the *DOE* as 'flow of blood, bleeding, hemorrhage', occurs in both the medical and penitential texts, and in each indicates a particular kind of menstrual disorder.[11] It occurs only once in the medical texts with reference to menstruation, in the *OEM*, referring elsewhere to nosebleeds, which suggests a specific kind of gushing blood rare in menstruation.[12] In *Leechdoms*, Thomas Cockayne refuses to translate this phrase when it refers to menstruation, and instead uncharacteristically chooses to use Latin in his translation of the Old English, saying 'ut menstrua fluant' instead.[13] Indeed, when this phrase appears with reference to nosebleeds, he has no compunction about translating it into English as 'blood running'.[14] *Blodryne* also occurs in the gospels, referring to the story of Veronica (unnamed in the gospels themselves), clearly referencing her 'blodryne twelf gear' ('bloodflow for twelve years').[15] Similarly, in Bede's account of the letters between Augustine of Canterbury and Pope Gregory I, Gregory refers to Veronica's excessive bleeding using *blodryne*, whereas in all other references to menstruation in this section of the letter he uses forms of *monaðaðl* or a phrase like 'blodes flownisse'.[16] Given Veronica's singular experience, the term *blodryne* does not signify regular menstruation, but rather disordered and excessive bleeding, and is used to indicate this rare condition.

Veronica's story of excessive menstruation and miraculous healing rely on notions of ritual pollution as well as physical disorder: she is a grand example of the impossibility of living one's life under the restrictions imposed by ritual impurity. In religious texts, including the penitentials, menstruation operates as a disabling factor resulting from impurity. Heide

Estes identifies menstruation as a kind of disability in Bede's *Ecclesiastical History*, arguing:

> Menstruation, like hunger and fever, is the result of original sin but is not sinful in itself. Yet the text's repetition that menstruation constitutes 'untrymness' creates a special category of infirmity particular to women, beyond the general states of hunger, etc. The characterization of menstruating women as 'untrym' suggests that the way later medieval as well as modern societies structurally disable women is also operative in Bede's account of menstruating women.[17]

Although Estes argues that menstruation itself is not sinful, the penitentials establish social prohibitions for women relative to their menstruating status, including prohibitions against receiving communion or having sex. At times, Old English language struggles to convey menstrual prohibitions more clearly articulated in Latin texts. In the case of the *Penitential of Theodore*, the menstrual prohibition becomes conflated with pre- and postnatal prohibitions, which can make it seem as if the menstrual prohibition has been excised from the text entirely.[18] The *DOE* suggests that the phrase *in gebyrdum monða tidum* means 'the time when nature ordains menstruation',[19] but the penitential removes the central 'monthly' element of the term. As Fulk and Jurasinski argue, *gebyrdtidum*

> always refers literally or metaphorically to the time of birth ... It is notable that in A 117 the translator plainly misconstrued or altered the meaning of 'menstruo tempore', taking it to refer to the month before childbirth. It is therefore possible that *gebyrdtidum*, though mistaken, is the more original reading in this instance. The following canon deals with postpartum cleansing, though the translator seems not to have comprehended this, taking it instead to refer to the end of menstruation.[20]

Thus, rather than expanding the vocabulary for menstruation as the *DOE* suggests, the compiler of the translation struggled to understand the Latin penitential and to find language in Old English for its precise designations about women's ritual uncleanness. In so doing, the author ultimately conflates all experiences of vaginal blood, and thereby technically fails to prohibit intercourse during menstruation.[21]

Of the Old English terms for menstruation, only *monaðadl* implies it is a fundamentally disordered process, connecting the idea of monthly occurrence with *adl*, meaning 'a disease, pain, a languishing sickness, consumption, morbus, languor'.[22] The exclusive Old English penitential term for menstruation, *monaðadl*, is used only for two purposes: to prohibit sex or to prohibit attendance at church.[23] First, in the *Old English Penitential*, it is deployed to prohibit sexual relations during menstruation: 'Swa hwýlc ceorl swa mid his wife in monaðadle hæme fæste xl nihta' ('Whichsoever man has sex with his menstruating woman is to fast forty nights').[24] Notably, the woman does not need cleansing or purification here, nor does she require penance for this action; only her partner seems to be defiled by sex during menstruation. Fulk and Jurasinski note that this kind of abstinence is required because of 'the belief that one suffered pollution from contact with blood or other bodily fluids'.[25] The implication is that a woman is fundamentally defiled by her own menstruation, and so it seems sex cannot further defile *her* at this time.[26]

The second use of the term confirms the polluted nature of the menstruating body, prohibiting not just what such a body can do, but where it can go. Little variation exists between the two manuscript versions of the *Old English Penitential*, which proscribe a menstruating woman from attending church or receiving the Eucharist: 'Wif in hire monaðadle cýricean né séce ne to husle ne ga naðer ne nunne ne læwede wif gif heo hit do fæste xx nihta' ('A woman in her monthly illness is not to approach the church or go to Eucharist, neither a nun nor a laywoman; if she does it she should fast twenty nights').[27] Unlike the sexual prohibition, this prohibition requires penance of the offending woman, but in a similar way it suggests her pollution of ritual and holy space and practices by virtue of the state of her menstruating body.[28] Thus, in the penitentials, menstruation, *monaðadl*, is configured as a contaminating illness in need of purification, a deficiency that only women can experience.

Bede also deploys *monaðadl* in his *Ecclesiastical History*, as a means of invoking the notion of ritual impurity in order to soften, if not disrupt, the idea entirely. In the eighth and ninth sections of the correspondence between Augustine of Canterbury and Pope Gregory I regarding correct practices for the newly converted English,

Augustine asks a series of questions about ritual impurity, and Gregory answers, making rather less of ritual purity than Augustine's questions seem to anticipate. Augustine's questions are derived from Levitican prohibitions, whereas Gregory's answers are often recast as shifting toward the New Law, wherein he 'recasts Augustine's construct of women as contaminating procreative organisms into creatures of God possessed of moral judgment. Defining menstruation as a consequence of the fall like hunger, thirst and weariness, Gregory does not supply the authoritative pronouncement demanded by Augustine's questions.'[29] Because Augustine's questions are fundamentally penitential in nature, Bede uses the penitential term 'monaþaðle' in translating the Latin. He retains it throughout the passage for both Augustine and Gregory, even when Gregory's response contradicts the penitentials outright, as he explicitly says:

> Hwæðre þæt wuufm mid þy heo þone gewunan þrowað monaþaðle, ne sceal heo bewered beon þæt heo mote in circan gongan; forðon seo oferflownis þæs gecyndes hire ne mæg in synne geteled beon, 7 þurh þæt þe heo þurh nead þrowað, nis þæt reht þæt heo sy bescyred from Godes circan ingonge.
>
> [Nevertheless the woman, when she endures her regular menstrual cycle, must not be forbidden from going into the church; because the overflowingness of her sex should not be tallied as a sin, and because she endures out of necessity, it is not right that she should be deprived of entering into God's church.][30]

Miller's translation falls back to the language of infirmity, changing the verb *þrowian* (to suffer or endure) into a noun, 'an affliction', thus pathologising the naming of the experience in a way that this part of the Old English text does not. My translation indicates Gregory's focus on the verb – to suffer or even just to endure – without identifying the experience of menstruation as itself an affliction. Gregory, in Bede's text, makes use of the same language as Augustine, but also redefines the nature of menstruation away from ritual impurity and into something that he newly identifies as the 'oferflownis þæs gecyndes' ('the overflowingness of her nature').[31] He reconfigures menstruation as natural, not polluting – a part of the nature or *gecynd* of woman, although he does ultimately identify menstruation as something that she 'nead þrowað' ('endures out of necessity').

In order to argue that menstruation is not a kind of pollution, Gregory aligns all menstruating women with Veronica, a woman in a constant state of hemorrhage. He thus conflates pathologised menstruation, *blodryne*, as discussed above, with *monaðadl* ('monthly illness'), a conflation that strikes me as particularly ironic because of course Veronica's illness is not monthly but, rather, constant. In order to 'liberat[e] Christian thought regarding menstruating and post-partal women from Levitical blood taboos', he must pathologise all menstruation.[32] He anticipates objection, saying (in Bede's rendering) 'Ac þu cwist nu: Heo nedde hire untrymnesse þæt he Cristes hrægle gehrine; þas wiif, bi þæm we sprecað, gelomlic gewuna getiið' ('But you say now, she because of her infirmity, was forced to touch Christ's clothing; the women of whom we speak, induced by repeated habit').[33] In this passage, what Veronica suffers is *untrymnesse* (weakness, sickness, illness, infirmity), whereas the menstruation of ordinary women is rather a repeated *gewuna*, a habit or custom, suggesting that Gregory anticipates that those who might disagree with him see menstruation not as an illness or affliction, but rather as a bad habit, often repeated. He argues against this point, stating explicitly just a few lines later that 'Hwæt wiifum heora monaðaðle blodes flownes bið untrymnis' ('Now for women the flowing of menstrual blood is an illness').[34] He has to identify menstruation as a sickness, in order to turn it from something unholy into something natural. Therefore he adds to the language of penance, *monaðadle*, by appending to it the phrase 'blodes flownes', the monthly illness of the flowing of blood, thereby using language to distinguish his understanding of menstruation from previous penitential approaches. Therefore, even as he argues against it, Gregory, particularly in the way his words are conveyed by Bede, preserves the notion of ritual impurity that we find in the other penitential texts.

While the language in even the least oppressive penitential texts designates menstruation as an impurity and illness, the language in the medical tradition describes physical symptoms without judgement. The medical texts compress the category of menstruation, both through its organisational annexing as a subset of general bloodflow, and through the narrow range of language for menstruation. They most often deploy the terms *monaðgecynd*, *monoðlican* and *flewsan*. Where the first two terms function euphemistically, referring to the cyclical nature of monthly menstruation, the latter applies a general term for the flowing of blood to describe in literal ways what menstruation is, with no need to disguise it in occlusive language. Taken as a whole, these terms work to identify medical needs dispassionately, divorcing taboo social perception from medical necessity.

Monaðgecynd combines the notion of monthliness with the idea of categories of identity in order to suggest that menstruation is a marker of identity or category, which is not to say that all women, and only women, menstruate. The combination of terms suggests that neither 'monthliness' nor 'kind' sufficiently indicates the idea of menstruation, but rather that they must be taken together. No dictionary yet accounts for the complex amalgamation of these two parts of the word.[35] *Monað* means monthly, but *gecynd* is a more complex term, whose definitions include 'nature', 'the established order of things' and 'the natural state', while the *DOE*'s definitions 6.a and 6.b refer to sex/gender and genitals, and 6.c to 'menstruation'.[36] Attesting that *gecynd* can mean menstruation when not connected to *monað* is a misreading of the text. The first occurrence of the term in *LBIII* says 'þe hire sio gecynd æt wære ahsa þæs æt þam wife' ('ask of the woman when her menstrual cycle might be').[37] The remedy is meant to treat obstructed menstruation: 'wifum sie forstanden hira monaþgecynd' ('for women, the obstruction of their menstruation').[38] In the first part of the quotation, 'gecynd' refers not to the menstruation (*monaðgecynd*), but rather to the *nature* – in other words, the timing of the woman's expected period. Similarly, a passage from *The Vercelli Homilies* VII, as cited in the *DOE* – 'for hwon wene ge, þæt wif swa sioce syn of hyre gecynde? ac hit is swa' ('why do you expect that women are so sick from their condition?') – is called into question by the *DOE* editors themselves, who suggest that *gecynd* might refer not to menstruation but to the third definition instead: 'nature, state, condition, position'.[39] Rather than taking *gecynd* to mean menstruation on its own, I suggest that pairing *monað* with *gecynd* indicates the connection between a monthly cycle and a woman's 'kind' or 'nature'. In other words, menses is an element of the category of woman. That *gecynd* also has definitions connected to the genitals of both sexes, as well as in definitions 9a and b – 'progeny, offspring' and 'power of procreation' respectively – locates it more fully in wider discourses of fertility and reproduction.[40]

Whereas *monaðgecynd* invokes the deep relation between identity and cycle, *monoðlican* removes the more complex term *gecynd* and replaces it with an adjectival ending, making the term at once clinical (in describing its repetitive regularity) and euphemistic (in not describing its physical properties). This term refers only to the monthliness of menstruation, and occurs in remedies that call up questions of time and timing. It occurs thirteen times, exclusively in the *OEH*, and in each instance refers to the desire of a woman to 'stir up' or summon menstruation that is occasionally described to be *forstanden*, obstructed. In certain ways, this term is closest to its Latin referent, *menstruum*, a term preferred and deployed frequently to gloss many of the Old English menstrual terms, as well as by later editors as a definition allowing them not to offer an English name for this taboo bodily process. Like *menstruus*, it means 'monthly', referring of course to the monthly occurrence of the shedding of the uterine lining. But because this term is so close to the Latin, conceptually, one wonders what ordinary women and speakers of Old English, not Latin, really called their own menstruation. As Elissa Stein and Susan Kim suggest, 'how did anyone talk about menstruation, you might wonder? The answer: rarely, and in the vaguest possible terms. Even today, advertisers and manufacturers tiptoe around the actual words, which are presumably too scary and horrible for our ladylike ears.'[41] In this way, any term meaning 'monthly' is a way of not identifying the fundamental and taboo part of the experience; it is a way of talking about timing, and not about blood.

As a strong contrast to words that focus on time and cycles, the term *flewsan* refers explicitly to discharge from any part of the body.[42] In the medical texts, *flewsa* is perhaps the least euphemistic of the common words for ordinary menstruation, indicating as it does the flow of fluids from the body. However, the fact that this term for menstruation is also used to describe any other kind of flow of fluids from the body might indicate a semantic connection with wounds or injuries rather than naturally occurring processes. Nosebleeds are a malady; blood flowing from a wound is an injury. According to the *DOE Web Corpus*, the term occurs approximately thirty-five times, seven of which are specific to menstruation. The *DOE* offers six definitions: (1) general flow/eye maladies; (2) 'Excessive discharge of semen'; (3) 'in women, excessive flow of blood or other discharge from the reproductive organs'; (4) flux from the belly/diarrhoea/dysentery; (5) 'referring to the woman diseased … for twelve years'; and (6) lust. Most of these definitions cite a single occurrence; only the definitions specific to menstruation (five occurrences listed from two texts) and flux from the belly (three occurrences listed from two texts) offer multiple occurrences, suggesting that though the term itself is a general one, it is used most frequently with reference to menstruation.

The function of individual words for menstruation is informed by context within remedies, within texts and textual traditions, within manuscripts, and within genres. In the penitential context, menstruation is a part of conversations about pollution and impurity; in the medical context, menstruation is a matter of reproductive health and treatment. While some of the language overlaps across these texts, the majority of the terms operate as anchored inside their distinct genres. The fact that there is not a unified name for the menstrual cycle across genres might suggest that menstruation is of little consequence to the authors of early medieval texts, or that it operates as a social taboo, or that it is a matter for discourse rather than textual preservation: we cannot fully know why. As with so many other features of early medieval women's lives, and despite their identification with this cyclical occurrence, its naming sits awkwardly inside the naming for more general categories – those for time, and those for the outflow of fluid. The frequency of remedies for menstruation, and its appearance in penitentials, do reveal that when Old English writers care about women's health concerns, what they care most about is regulating menstruation, even if they cannot agree on what it should be called.

Remedies for stopping flow

As my discussion of the problem of naming makes clear, the question of and orientation toward menstruation are not straightforward in early medieval culture. In the following sections, I divide remedies for menstruation into two categories: those for stopping an unwanted flow, and those for provoking a missing flow. Ultimately the combination of formulaic language and desired outcomes stated in the remedies signify common functions. Within each of these two categories, a variety of complications or conditions informs the need for the result. What we cannot tell from these remedies is what lies behind the diagnostic question 'How do I make my flow stop?' or 'What should I do if my period is late?' A woman might wish to stop or start her flow for a variety of reasons, and so remedies that suggest the same result might not necessarily treat the same condition. In fact, the lack of medical knowledge about individual conditions, particularly with respect to the remedies for stopping excessive flow, means that most remedies in this category follow humoral ideas of drying up excessive moisture, or blocking up a too-leaky body. These remedies often use the formulaic phrase *wið wifa flewsan* ('for a woman's flow') to signal their intent, even when the remedies themselves do not clearly identify the hoped-for result. Given the squeamish nineteenth-century scholarly response to menstrual remedies, contemporary scholars often struggle to determine what these remedies seek to treat, but the formulaic language can help us to determine common maladies, even when other parts of the remedy offer little information.

The remedies for stopping flow most frequently use the term *flewsan* to identify the malady they wish to treat, but only offer remediation for the symptom, excessive bleeding. Although they do not explicitly employ the language of humoral medicine, they prescribe remedies that operate within its ideologies, suggesting implicitly and sometimes explicitly that excessive menstruation is simply a form of wetness in need of drying up, or that the female body is a leaky vessel that requires closing.[43] Remedies based on these principles cannot have been successful, and might indeed in a number of cases have caused harm. A likely culprit for this kind of bleeding is menorrhagia (heavy menstrual bleeding), a condition that affects approximately 30 per cent of the current population of women of reproductive age and is linked to a number of resulting and underlying conditions from anaemia to polycystic ovaries.[44] The desire for the cessation of a flow indicates a kind of disordered menstruation, one that is painful or dangerous, particularly to women already living in nutritional deficit and who are iron-deficient, and who explicitly might have sought menstrual regulation to promote fertility.

The two remedies from the *OEH* using comfrey both employ the term *flewsan*, and suggest in context that the goal of the remedy is to bind up the flow of liquid through an internal mechanism. The remedies offer only minor variation in the desired result of the remedy, suggesting that they were meant to treat the same, or at least a similar, malady. Despite variant given names (*galluc confirma* and *Halswyrt/sinfitus albus*), Anne Van Arsdall identifies both herbs as comfrey.[45] In fact, both remedies require the same preparation, using almost identical language. Both call for someone to 'cnuca to swyþe smalon duste' ('pound it into a fine powder') and 'syle drincan on wine' ('give it to drink in wine').[46] The only notable difference in language between these two remedies appears in the results: where 60.1 suggests the 'flewsa ætstandeþ' ('stops'), 128.1 says that the 'flewsan gewrið' ('is bound up'). While the result seems basically the same, the latter gives more specific language for the means by which such a flow might be ended: that its source will be 'bound', or 'tied up'. We know, then, that the binding of the source was believed possible by means of a consumed herbal beverage, which suggests a malady that is understood as no more than extra liquid that can be internally stopped.[47]

Just as the language of binding up menstruation emphasises the way in which it is constituted by the flow of liquid, so too the remedies using nettle and yarrow in *OEH* focus on the liquid nature of *flewsan*, thus indicating their shared desired outcome. While the remedy for nettle suggests in simple terms that it is 'wið wifes flewsan' ('for a woman's flow'), the remedy for yarrow offers slightly more information: 'Gif wif of ðam gecyndelican flewsan þæs wætan þoligen' ('if a woman suffers a flow of moisture from the genitals').[48] Van Arsdall translates the passage 'If a woman is troubled by fluid flowing from her sexual organ', where 'flewsan' operates as a verb, 'flowing'. She explains this choice, commenting on the distinction between the Latin original and the Old English version, saying 'the Old English original does not say this is specifically menstrual (*monaðlic*) flux; from the Old English, it could be merely a discharge'.[49] On the contrary, I argue that it is important to understand this word as a noun, parallel with most other remedies meant to stop excessive menstrual flow, where the adjectival *monaðlic* is neither necessary nor regularly employed. In fact, she clearly identifies the remedy for nettle as 'for a woman's menses', despite its use of the word *flewsan* without any adjectival modifier. The choice is further supported by the clearly menstrual nature of the original Latin. The amalgamation of possible nouns (*gecyndelican, flewsan, wætan*) might easily have resulted from a monastic scribe scrambling to convey the sense of the passage with a barrage of vaguely menstrual/liquid terms. Menstruation's affiliation with freely flowing liquid then contributes to the sense of how to treat it – by binding up, stoppering or even drying.

As a further testament to their treatment of a parallel malady, the remedies for nettle and yarrow both treat menstrual excess by simply attempting to dry it up. The *OEH* remedy using yarrow seeks to end a flow of menstrual liquid through heat-induced evaporative strategies, suggesting that sitting on a boiled yarrow plant will 'ealne þone wæ(t)an of hyre æþme heo gewrið' ('dry up all the wetness with vapor'),[50] while the remedy using nettle calls for use of pounded nettle mixed with honey spread onto wet wool, with which a practitioner should 'smyre ðonne þa geweald mid þam læcedom, ond syþþan hyne þam wife gesyle þat heo hyne hyre under gelecge. þy sylfan dæge hyt þone flewsan beluceð' ('smear the genitals with the medication, and afterwards give it to the woman, so that she can lay it under herself. That same day, it will stop the flow').[51] Both remedies employ the same kind of metaphor for the desired outcome: the former claims to dry up or even wrap around, 'gewrið', the 'moisture', by means of a hot vapour, whereas the latter proposes to 'lock up', 'beluceð', the flow as quickly as possible. While the outcome of the remedies here is clear (drying up or locking up the flow), it is only the symptom, the *flewsan*, that they treat, believing that symptom to reveal an imbalance of humours as the cause.[52] These remedies therefore articulate and confirm notions about women's leaky bodies as vessels in need of locking or binding up by external forces, those provided by men as authors of these texts, who will find the means of 'locking' and 'binding', an apt metaphor for their treatment of women's lives as well as their bodies.

The diagnostic body and the matter of menstruation 49

Like the vapour that locks up a leaky body, smoke, too, can be applied to a body exhibiting an excessive flow of blood. This remedy in *LBIII* is meant to resolve the problem of a flow that is 'to swiþe' ('too strong') by applying smoke to the genitals (performed while the patient is clothed) with coal-heated horse dung: 'Gif wife to swiþe offlowe sio monað gecynd. genim niwe horses tord lege on hate gleda læt reocan swiþe betweoh þa þeoh up under þæt hrægl þæt se mon swæte swiþe' ('If for a women the monthly cycle flows out too much: take fresh horse manure, lay it on hot embers; let it smoke forcefully between the thighs up under the clothing, so that the person sweats heavily').[53] As in the previous example, the focus remains on humoral wetness, where the smoking does not merely dry off the symptom of externalised fluid, but rather the heat directed at her thighs invokes a whole-body effluvia, draining the body of excess fluid and thus solving the imbalance of humours. Here, sweat and menstruation are treated as originating with the same internal malady, a commonality that strangely disrupts the connection between regulated menstruation and fertility in real terms, if not in humoral ones. Further, this treatment is clearly unpleasant, exacerbating the abject nature of the menstrual body, treating abject liquid with abject smoke.

In contrast to this smoking treatment, the medical tradition's response to postpartum bleeding – and the language it uses to identify such bleeding – is quite different, indicating a distinction in treatment relative to cause, and suggesting that the previous treatments would not have been used universally to stop *all* kinds of gynaecological bloodflow, or that they all would have been understood as relative to the humours. In a practical sense, it might be difficult but also dangerous to treat the genitals of a woman who has just given birth with smoking horse dung. Instead, this postpartum remedy calls for the eating and drinking of herbs, and does not use any of the terms used in the remedies for excessive menstruation: 'Gif [hio] blede to swiþe æfter þam beorþre nioþowearde clatan wyl on meolce sele etan and supan þæt wos' ('If [she] bleeds too much after the birth: boil the lower part of goosegrass in milk, give it [to her] to eat and sip the liquid').[54] The woman's discharge is not fitted into the category of *flewsa* here, but rather she is described as actively bleeding. Whereas the previous remedy is concerned with the 'flowing out too quickly of her *monthly nature*', this remedy has no compunction about identifying the fluid as blood. It seems fair to say that in so doing, the writer understands that what is flowing out derives from a dangerous wound, rather than a cyclical biological process. However, like the other remedies in this section, it offers no clear articulation of the expected result. Will the bleeding stop? Slow? Lighten? Will this remedy offer pain relief or somehow staunch a haemorrhage? The remedy responds to a frequent problem, but offers frustratingly little information about the results it might produce to help a woman in urgent need.

Taken as a whole, these remedies to stop flow wish to make absent the all-too-troubling presence of unwanted and excessive bleeding using a consistent pattern of language to indicate menstrual excess as opposed to other kinds of genital bleeding. They rely on humoral principles that, at best, provide consumable treatments that would have relied on the placebo effect for success. However, at worst, they degrade and make abject the bodies of suffering women, confirming for both the female patient and the persons offering and applying treatment the grotesque nature of a body that is characterised by its regular capacity to flow beyond its limits. The language of the response to stopping an excessive or unwanted flow is centred in the squeezing shut of a body that is too open, harnessing and choking up the taboo blood that is also understood to be a necessary component of reproductive viability. Even in a medical tradition that evades the sin-based penitential language for menstruation, women's bodies, overflowing with liquids, are set up as out of control and in need of authoritative clerical intervention. It is only by means of this figure of knowledge and authority that such an unruly body can be constricted and made to behave.

Remedies for provoking flow

If the reasons a woman might wish to stop an excessive menstrual flow are obvious, the reasons for starting one become more complicated. Monica Green suggests that even after the increase of surgical interventions for complex births in the sixteenth century, 'the defining tasks for the physician remained his involvement with regulating women's menstruation, ensuring fertility, and addressing other internal diseases of the female genitalia'.[55] Although Green's work is based on later medicine from continental Europe, the early medieval English texts demonstrate an enduring focus on menstruation and fertility. Remedies for menstruation, stopping it or starting it, are generally invested in the maintenance of fertility. A woman who seeks to provoke menstruation may do so because she wishes to regulate and promote her fertility by restoring a missing or irregular cycle. However, remedies for the restoration of a menstrual cycle also provide means of preventing conception. Because of the expanded timeline for conception, discussed in Chapter 4, these remedies for restoration of menstruation function in a way that in contemporary terms we might identify as early abortion. Pregnancy is not always welcome, and the desire to provoke a flow might have as much to do with avoiding pregnancy as with enabling it.

Although the remedies are rarely explicit about the reason for provoking a flow, their patterns of language may help distinguish the problems they are meant to address. In the remedies, menstruals may be *astyrian* (stirred),[56] or *gecigde* (called forth or summoned), or they may be identified as *forstanden* (absent).[57] Remedies that do not identify a symptom may be just doing their due diligence in offering some remedies for women. Intentionally or otherwise, remedies that offer women a means of provoking a menstrual flow, or that suggest that such a thing can be done, disclose a truth about women's lives. Even if such a remedy might not be efficacious, it shows that a woman might *desire* to determine for herself not only when she menstruates, but also, as a direct result, when or if she reproduces. It represents a more flexible notion of conception through language that might even appear to contemporary readers as coded. These remedies for provoking flow do not make use of the kinds of humoral medicine present in the remedies for stopping excessing flow. Instead, they often employ variations on known abortifacients (substances that induce abortion) and emmenagogues (substances that increase menstrual flow). Such remedies point to the potential of women to desire and perhaps attempt to operate control over their own fertility, stirring or summoning not just a regular cycle, but in some instances preventing or dislodging conception.

By leaving out details, remedies for provoking flow do not specify why a woman might wish to summon her menstrual cycle. Indeed, most remedies provide little information, serving as part of a long list of potential uses for herbs, particularly in *OEH*, as is the case for bishop's weed: 'eac hyt ða monoðlican forð gecigeþ' ('also it summons forth the menstruals').[58] Similarly, *OEH* proposes the use of shepherd's purse, St John's wort and German iris to 'stir up' menses, with iris treating even long-term amenorrhoea: 'hit þæra wifa monoliðlican astyreð þeah hy ær langæ forlætene wæron' ('it stirs the women's menses, even though they might have been absent for a long time').[59] The vagueness of this final phrase might be an attempt to treat a wide range of women, from those with nutritional deficits, to those who might have been nursing a child, or those having borne a series of children over a number of years thus suppressing menstruation – even to those, the remedy seems to suggest, past menopause. If we read this remedy as indicative of the category of 'stirring' as a whole, it suggests an affiliation with promoting or restoring fertility. Alternatively, it would be unorthodox, although not impossible, to infer that menses *forlætan* (absent) might be those missing due to an unwanted pregnancy, particularly given the wide semantic range of the word, which here suggests interruption of a natural flow, but elsewhere means 'to allow', 'to release' or even 'to abandon'.[60] Therefore, *forlætan* is a word that can be its own opposite (both allowing and abandoning), and so it expresses rather poetically the problem of the present-absence of a menstrual cycle, one that a woman either might wish returned so that it might soon be absent, or one that a woman might just wish returned. The absence of expressed motive leaves space for a range of possibilities that may or may not have been understood by the men writing these texts.

The language in the *OEM* remedy, which calls for a more elaborate ritual, implies even more strongly a contraceptive impulse, informed further by its rhetorical placement following a remedy using similar methods to 'cleanse' or purge a woman.[61] Whereas previous remedies invoke stirring of the menses by compounds, this one sounds more like a ritual command for a rush of blood, and it relies on the woman herself to perform these ablutions proactively and independently:

> Eft gif heo wylle þæt ðæt hyre blodryne cyme to, cembe eft hyre heafod under morbeame, and þæt feax þe on þam cambe cleofige, somnige and do on anne telgran ðe sy adune gecyrred, and gesamnige eft; þæt hyre byþ læcedom.
>
> [Again, if she wants to have her flow back: let her comb again her head under the mulberry tree, and gather the hair that sticks to the comb and place it on a twig that is turned downwards, and afterwards gather it; this will be her remedy.][62]

It is the woman who must locate the tree, and must comb, place and gather her own hair. Her remedy is entirely contained in her own body and action, in contrast with most other remedies, which seem to be compounded for or enacted upon women. The terminology here and in *Bald* – *blodryne* and *blodsihtan* respectively – suggests something rather more gushing than a simple return to a regular cycle. Such a rush of blood (notably *not* described as a *flewsan* or more typical menstrual language) seems to be something more akin to cleansing of excess tissue, or, perhaps, abortion.[63] These remedies that wish to provoke menstruation, then, may be more complex than just attempting to assist and facilitate conception. They may be, in part, about forestalling it.

While these remedies leave open the potential for reproductive control by what they do not say, only one remedy explicitly comments on what might be expelled from a woman's body with a returned menstrual cycle, establishing its function as an abortifacient.[64] The *OEH* lists a second function for wallflower, beyond its use to 'call forth' menses; by means of pounding the wallflower with wine or honey, and consuming it *or* applying it to the genitals, it will both 'stir' the menstruals, *and* lead out *tudder*, offspring: 'Wyþ ða monoðlican to astyrigenne … hyt þa monoðlican astyreþ ond þæt tudder of þam cwiðan gelædeþ' ('for the stirring of menstruation … It stirs menstruation and brings out the foetus from the womb').[65] This remedy is explicitly NOT about helping with a difficult labour, or expelling a *deadboren* – stillborn – child. While there are remedies that are explicitly for stillbirths, we can infer that this is not one of them, if we are attentive to the language. It declares its purpose not once, but twice: to stir up menses. While giving birth (to either a live or a dead child) leads to bleeding, it does not lead to bleeding of the *monaþlican*, monthly sort. Rather, if a *tudder* is being brought out from the womb in the service of reviving a monthly flow, it might well be as a result of either circumventing conception or causing abortion.[66] This remedy demonstrates the potential of remedies, particularly those provoking flow, to serve women in ways that might be contrary to the desires of the patriarchy at large, hidden in plain sight and resting on the abject nature of menstruation.[67]

All of the medical manuscripts offer remedies that might be understood to be abortifacients, but the framing of these remedies as being for the restoration of menstruation locates them in a different register. While the inclusion of such remedies in manuscripts transcribed by monks or nuns might be a case of hiding such preparations in plain sight, it more probably represents a different understanding of conception. Like the remedy from the *OEH*, this remedy in *LBIII* suggests a return to menstruation connected to the prevention of conception or pregnancy: here, the woman's flow is depicted as having been 'obstructed' by something: 'Wiþ þon þe wifum sie forstanden hira monaþgecynd' ('In case a woman's menstruation is obstructed'),[68] perhaps a tumour, but also perhaps a foetus; the indeterminacy serves to open rather than foreclose on the possibility. This elaborate remedy calls for boiling, drinking, bathing and then bathing while drinking, but all of this must take place in alignment with the woman's expected menstrual period: 'Þu scealt simle þam wife bæþ wyrcean and drenc sellan on þa ilcan tid. þe hire sio gecynd æt wære ahsa þæs æt þam wife' ('You must always make the bath and give the drink for the woman at the same time as her menstrual period might be. You must ask this time of the woman').[69] This remedy requires a great deal of labour, and very specific elements that must occur in a particular order and for an extended duration. The timing of the remedy relative to the expected timing of the woman's menstrual cycle suggests that it seeks to prevent conception, and perhaps aims to avoid a missed menstrual cycle at all. According to Marijane Osborn, brooklime and centaury were known abortifacients, and mugwort was used both to facilitate birth and as an abortifacient.[70] That the remedy is to be repeated accounts for potential variations in potency, probably preventing too strong a dose, which might be dangerously toxic. These variations in repetition might also be related to just

The diagnostic body and the matter of menstruation 55

how long a menstrual cycle might have been absent: the longer the absence might call for a higher dose of these many collected herbal concoctions to be both consumed and applied.

If these remedies for provoking menstruation were simply an inverse mirror of the remedies for stopping excess menstruation, we might expect to see a humoral response akin to the idea of drying out what is too liquid. Perhaps bathing the woman participates in this humoral idea, but paired as it is with herbal ingredients that provoke known abortifacient processes, that principle does not seem to be the main notion here. Instead, these remedies for provoking menstruation rely on a woman's own knowledge of her menstrual cycle. She has to know and provide specific information in order for the timing to be correct and the remedy to succeed. The remedies require her to consult with a knowledgeable physician who will try to provoke her cycle at the correct time – not too early and, most importantly, not too late. If a woman is missing a period (and she knows when it ought to arrive), then it seems likely that she may be pregnant. If her periods are irregular or missing, then she is unlikely to know when her period should begin. While not all remedies for provoking menstruation indicate exactly the same practices and outcomes, several do indicate a complex set of motives for seeking to bring on a menstrual cycle.

Conclusions: Menstruation, fertility and reproduction

Menstruation is a necessary process for typical unmedicated reproductive health. With few other diagnostic methods, medieval practitioners could probably tell very little about a woman's gynaecological health or her ability to achieve and sustain a pregnancy. Therefore, it comes as no surprise that the greatest proportion of remedies for women focus on menstruation, either in its excess or its lack. While diagnostically crucial, socially menstruation occupies a troubled niche in medieval discussions of women's bodies. It is at once a taboo, a polluting liquid, a disorder, an illness and a regular occurrence aligned with moon phases. It signals reproductive health and fertility, and indicates danger in its excess. It is at once overdetermined and underexamined. Even now, menstruation receives far less scholarly attention and funding than erectile dysfunction,[71] and many women lack knowledge about their own bodies and menstruation. While Old English medical remedies and penitentials can give us some sense of the early medieval understanding of menstruation, never do we hear about it from women themselves: the closest we can come is in the implied questions that both remedy and penitential suggest.

We cannot be certain that women ever actually accessed or used these menstrual remedies. Instead, such remedies reflect beliefs and ideas about women's bodies and reproduction, some of which derive from classical tradition, some from local practices, and all of which are framed by the people in institutions that produced such texts. They participate in the textual construction of women's bodies. Like the penitentials, which offer spiritual diagnoses and treatments, the medical texts too offer their own form of diagnosis and remediation. They construct the idea of a female body, perhaps one that is less shameful than the one produced by the penitentials. Even so, some of the practical concerns and requirements for and of women's reproductive bodies exist within these pages, pushing both transcriber and translator to interact with unfamiliar body parts, distasteful effluvia and taboo procedures. Medical texts include information meant to regulate not only menses but potentially also reproduction. Whether or not the people who transcribed and used these texts understood this language, and whether or not they were ever used in England to treat women, the texts both set forth and conceal the potential for women to control their own reproduction. The trick of remedies is that they are not individual; they exist not to serve one person, but to serve a class united by similar suffering; they respond to the needs of women at large and turn the sufferers of individual maladies into a community bound by common physical experience. These remedies give us a small window into the experience of a woman attempting to regulate her reproductive potential in a textual culture that rarely acknowledges women, and that depicts their bodies even more rarely.

Notes

1 Beck, Julie, 'Women Astronauts: To Menstruate or Not to Menstruate', *The Atlantic* (21 April 2016), www.theatlantic.com/health/archive/2016/04/menstruating-in-space/479229/ (accessed 25 July 2022).

2 UN News, 'Break Taboo around Menstruation, Act to End "Disempowering" Discrimination, Say UN experts' (5 March 2019), https://news.un.org/en/story/2019/03/1034131#:~:text=A%20group%20of%20seven%20United,to%20end%20%E2%80%9Cdisempowering%E2%80%9D%20discrimination (accessed 25 July 2022).
3 United Nations Population Fund, 'Menstruation and Human Rights – Frequently Asked Questions' (May 2022), www.unfpa.org/menstruationfaq (accessed 25 July 2022).
4 Babbar, Karan, Jennifer Martin, Josephine Ruiz, Ateeb Ahmad Parray and Marni Sommer, 'Menstrual Health Is a Public Health and Human Rights Issue', *The Lancet: Public Health* (27 October 2021), DOI: 10.1016/S2468-2667(21)00212-7 (accessed 17 July 2023).
5 *OEH*, in John P. Niles and Maria D'Aronco (eds and trans), *Anglo-Saxon Medical Texts*, Vol. I, *The Old English Herbal, Lacnunga, and Other Texts*, Dumbarton Oaks Medieval Library (Cambridge, MA: Harvard University Press, 2023), p. 210 (90.16).
6 Przemysław Tyszka, 'The Conceptualisation of Men and Women by the Authors of Penitentials', in Anndrzej Pleszczynski, Joanna Sobiesiak, Michał Tomaszek and Przemysław Tyszka (eds), *Imagined Communities Constructing Collective Identities in Medieval Europe* (Leiden: Brill, 2018), pp. 222–43 (p. 224).
7 Erik Wade, '*Pater* Don't Preach: Byzantine Theology, Female Sexuality, and Histories of Global Encounter in the "English" *Pænitentiale Theodori*', *The Medieval Globe*, 4.2 (2018): 1–28 (p. 12). See also Christine Fell, with Cecily Clark and Elizabeth Williams, *Women in Anglo-Saxon England and the Impact of 1066* (London: British Museum Publications, 1984), especially pp. 56–73. In this chapter, Fell discusses issues of punishment for sexual behaviours, but uses mainly the laws of Cnut and Æþelbert, sermons, and even poems as evidence. The closest she comes in this chapter is to say 'there are other types of evidence that offer a less attractive picture. Homilies and letters from the pens of clergy and missionaries thunder against polygamy and incest. It is a range of evidence I find difficult to assess' (p. 71).
8 Wade, '*Pater* Don't Preach', pp. 12–13.
9 Ibid., p. 8.
10 Research that is focused explicitly on the subject is, however, extremely limited. While menstruation appears in discussion for both genres, little scholarship takes it as a primary subject. One of the only pieces to do so is Charles T. Wood, 'The Doctors' Dilemma: Sin, Salvation, and the Menstrual Cycle in Medieval Thought', *Speculum: A Journal of Medieval Studies*, 56.4 (1981), 710–27.

11 Joseph Bosworth, 'blód-ryne', in *An Anglo-Saxon Dictionary Online*, ed. Thomas Northcote Toller, Christ Sean and Ondřej Tichy (Prague: Faculty of Arts, Charles University, 2014), https://bosworthtoller.com/4726 (accessed 23 December 2023); 'blodryne', in Angus Cameron, Ashley Crandell Amos, Antonette diPaolo Healey et al. (eds), *Dictionary of Old English: A to I Online* (Toronto: Dictionary of Old English Project, 2018) (*DOE*), https://tapor.library.utoronto.ca/doe/ (accessed 23 December 2023).

12 *OEM*, in Niles and D'Aronco, *Anglo-Saxon Medical Texts*, Vol. I, p. 374 (2.3). The *OEM* uses the term 'blodryne' five times, with the other four occurrences referring to general bleeding, or, most commonly, nosebleeds. It occurs a total of twenty-one times in the *DOE Web Corpus*.

13 Thomas Oswald Cockayne, *Leechdoms, wortcunning, and starcraft of early England. Being a collection of documents, for the most part never before printed, illustrating the history of science in this country before the Norman Conquest*, 3 vols (London: Longman, Green, Longman, Roberts and Green, 1864–66), Vol. II, p. 333.

14 Ibid., Vol. II, pp. 347, 349 (twice in the same passage) and 353.

15 Matthew, Mark and Luke use close variations of this phrase, cited in the *DOE Web Corpus*. Cambridge, Corpus Christi College (CCC), MS 140: Skeat 1871–87, 8–134; W. W. Skeat, *The Four Gospels in Anglo-Saxon, Northumbrian, and Old Mercian Versions* (Cambridge: Cambridge University Press, 1871–87).

16 Bede, *The Old English Version of Bede's Ecclesiastical History of the English People*, ed. and trans. Thomas Miller, Early English Text Society (Oxford: Oxford University Press, 1959 (1890)), p. 78, line 11.

17 'Untrym' means weakness or illness. Heide Estes, 'Menstruation, Infirmity, and Religious Observance from Ecclesiastical History', in Cameron Hunt McNabb (ed.), *Medieval Disability Sourcebook* (Goleta, CA: Punctum Books, 2020), pp. 341–44 (p. 342).

18 R. D. Fulk and Stefan Jurasinski (eds), *The Old English Canons of Theodore*, Early English Text Society (Oxford: Oxford University Press, 2012), XIV.17.

19 Angus Cameron, Ashley Crandell Amos, Antonette diPaolo Healey et al. (eds), *Dictionary of Old English: A to I Online* (Toronto: Dictionary of Old English Project, 2018), https://tapor.library.utoronto.ca/doe/ (accessed 23 December 2023), as referencing the passage from Theodore A.113.

20 Fulk and Jurasinski, *The Old English Canons*, p. 58.

21 'The translator renders this statement as a prohibition against intercourse during the final month of pregnancy rather than during menstruation. [*Pœnitentiale Theodori*] (I, xiv, 18) and many other penitentials forbade conjugal relations before the ritual purification of women after childbirth ... for the same reason that abstinence was required during menstruation – the belief that one suffered pollution from contact with blood or other bodily fluids' (ibid., pp. 60–1), and finally, 'The commitment of the translator to this eccentric rendering means that traditional restrictions against intercourse during menstruation, conventional in the collections to which he may have had access, are ultimately absent from his own' (p. 61). Pierre Payer also clearly notes variation in terms of the length of penance for menstrual intercourse in the *Canons of Theodore*, indicating that the Latin text discusses this prohibition in multiple instances; Pierre J. Payer, *Sex and the Penitentials: The Development of a Sexual Code 550–1150* (Toronto: University of Toronto Press, 1984), p. 25.

22 Bosworth–Toller effaces the referent of the term, generalising it to mean 'a disease that occurs at intervals of a month', implying that any person might experience such a disease, while all of the occurrences of it are explicitly specific to menstruation. The choice of language here is generally used as translation for Latin 'sanguine menstruo', or 'tempore menstruo', which appear as glosses in two out of the three occurrences: in *The Old English Penitential*, also known as Pseudo-Egberti, found respectively in Oxford, Bodleian Library, MS Junius 121, s. XI¾, Worcester (Ker 338; Gneuss 644), 89a; and Oxford, Bodleian Library, MS Junius 121, s. XI¾; Worcester (Ker 338; Gneuss 644), 93a. Cited, with regrets on account of his misogynistic statements about feminist principles and women, from Allen Frantzen (ed), *Anglo-Saxon Penitentials: A Cultural Database, Oxford, Bodleian Library, Junius 121, s. XI¾; Worcester, 93b. X14.07.01*, www.anglo-saxon.net/penance/index.php?p=JUNIUS_93b (accessed 16 July 2023).

23 *Monaðadl* appears four times in the penitentials, one of which is a header for a section 'be monaðadles hæmede & be oþrum unrihthæmede' (about intercourse during menstruation and other fornication); Pseudo-Egberti, CCC, MS 190, 18(16), referenced in *DOE Web Corpus*.

24 From Frantzen, *Anglo-Saxon Pentitentials* (Oxford, Bodleian Library, MS Junius 121, s. XI¾, Worcester (Ker 338; Gneuss 644), 89a).

25 Fulk and Jurasinski, *Old English Canons*, pp. 60–1.

26 It is possible that this is a result of humoral medicine, and the notion that through her menstruation a woman is purged of 'noxious blood'. See Elissa Stein and Susan Kim, *Flow: The Cultural History of Menstruation* (New York: St Martin's Griffin, 2009), p. 7, although they also note that 'many religions and cultures cleverly devised ritualized cleansing ceremonies to regularly purge women of their monthly impurities' (p. 81). Erik Wade remarks: 'According to the [*Pœnitentiale Theodori*], women are not responsible for sexual sins committed with men: the canons prescribe penances for men who commit sins with women, but not for the women … There is little suggestion that a woman actually sins in most of the sexual acts that a man might commit with her. Those sins are considered to be his failings. This principle stands in stark contrast to the misogynistic tradition of the later Middle Ages, which typically treated women as the instigators of male sexual sins.' Wade, '*Pater* Don't Preach', p. 17.

27 From Frantzen, *Anglo-Saxon Penitentials* (Oxford, Bodleian Library, MS Junius 121, s. XI¾, Worcester (Ker 338; Gneuss 644), 93a), with the other occurrence being Oxford, Bodleian Library, MS Laud Misc. 482, s. XImed, Worcester (Ker 343; Gneuss 656), 17b. See also Stefan Jurasinski, *The Old English Penitentials and Anglo-Saxon Law* (Cambridge: Cambridge University Press, 2015), p. 81.

28 Wade says 'But the canons do expect women to do penance for entering a church or taking communion while menstruating, demonstrating that women are held responsible for managing their impurity in other aspects of their lives, but not with respect to sexual acts with their husbands'; Wade, '*Pater* Don't Preach', p. 18.

29 Stephanie Hollis, *Anglo-Saxon Women and the Church: Sharing a Common Fate* (Woodbridge: Boydell Press, 1992), p. 25. Rob Meens says 'It was Augustine's "own prior cultural construct", trained as he was by reading the early Fathers and the Bible (including, of course, Leviticus), that made him choose questions about ritual purity among others, to refer to the pope. His supposed lack of experience in pastoral care, due to his monastic upbringing, would have been another factor' (Rob Meens, 'A Background to Augustine's Mission to Anglo-Saxon England', *Anglo-Saxon England*, 23 (1994), 5–17 (p. 11). Though Hollis thus gives credit to Augustine's own upbringing and the ecclesiastical traditions behind it, she strongly suggests that it was early medieval English attitudes that, like similar Judeo-Christian beliefs, conspired to prevent 'carnal profanation of the sacred' (Hollis, *Anglo-Saxon Women*, p. 25). Erik Wade also notes: 'The answers that women received from Archbishop Theodore in response to their inquiries often have no clear antecedent in previous penitentials or in

English lawcodes, both of which tend to focus on male sexual acts. Hollis notes that the [*Pœnitentiale Theodori*] differs from the *Libellus responsionum* – Pope Gregory's answers to the theological questions of Augustine ... by providing little room for individual women to judge the appropriateness of their actions by themselves. For example, where the *Libellus* recommends that menstruating women not enter a church unless they themselves judge it spiritually necessary, the [*Pœnitentiale Theodori*] flatly forbids them from doing so under any circumstances' (Wade, '*Pater* Don't Preach', p. 13).

30 Bede, *Ecclesiastical History*, ed. and trans. Miller, p. 78. Miller translates the passage thus: 'Yet the woman, while menstruous, shall not be prohibited from going to church, for the natural overflow may not be counted as her sin, and it is not right that she should be cut off from entering God's church through a necessary affliction' (p. 79).

31 *Oferflown* occurs only thirteen times in the *DOE Web Corpus*, and this seems to be the only occurrence that refers to menstruation.

32 Becky R. Lee, 'The Purification of Women after Childbirth: A Window onto Medieval Perceptions of Women', *Florilegium*, 14 (1995–96), 43–55 (p. 46). Lee suggests that Franz is overly optimistic here, not because Gregory is not attempting to liberate women from the problem of pollution, but because of the way postpartal prohibitions continue in the tradition after Gregory.

33 Bede, *Ecclesiastical History*, ed. and trans. Miller, pp. 78–9. It should be noted that Veronica remains nameless in this passage, although she is generally accepted to be the referent. Indeed, in one of the three extant versions of this text her name is excised altogether. See Mary Swan, 'Remembering Veronica in Anglo-Saxon England', in Elaine Treharne (ed.), *Writing Gender and Genre in Medieval Literature* (London: D. S. Brewer, 2002), pp. 19–40 (p. 34).

34 Bede, *Ecclesiastical History*, ed. and trans. Miller, pp. 78–89.

35 This term occurs only four times in the corpus of Old English, and only in *LBIII*. Bosworth–Toller defines the term only through its Latin referent, *menstruum*, perpetuating a perhaps unsurprising nineteenth-century discomfort with the leaky bodies of women. The *DOE* has not yet reached the letter 'm', and so has no relevant information.

36 The *DOE Web Corpus* lists 618 occurrences of this term, with the vast preponderance of them referring to the general ideas of 'nature' and 'kind'.

37 Cockayne, *Leechdoms*, Vol. II, pp. 330/332 (3.38.2).

38 Ibid., Vol. II, p. 330 (3.38.1).

39 Samantha Zacher's edition includes the Latin parallel, 'num ex conditione sexus tantum' (surely not from the cause of their sex alone),

in 'The Source of Vercelli VII: An Address to Women', in Samantha Zacher and Andy Orchard (eds), *New Readings in the Vercelli Book* (Toronto: University of Toronto Press, 2009), pp. 98–149 (p. 136). The phrase that precedes this parallel passage clarifies that the text is discussing not menstruation, but rather the nature of women: 'From what cause or from what kind of reason do you think that women are so weak and feeble?' (the answer: 'from their lifestyle and upbringing' (p. 137), including the use of fancy oil and perfumes while lying around in bed). It is not impossible to infer that a woman might be made sick by her menstruation, but that is not the case in this passage. Given the flawed nature of both listed passages, I suggest that menstruation is not an accurate definition for *gecynd*.

40 Another word that has been mischaracterised by contemporary resources is *monaðseoc*, a word that means 'moon-sick'. Jane Roberts, Christian Kay and Lynne Grundy, *A Thesaurus of Old English* (Leiden: Brill, 2000), suggest *monaðseoc* as an alternative term for menstruation, but the idea of moon-sickness, though perhaps originally grounded in the connection between monthly cycles and emotional instability, is not fundamentally connected to menstruation, nor is it experienced solely by women. Animals and humans are treated for it in the remedies, but it does not appear in any medical texts as referring to menstruation. While we can see these struggles to identify the limits and language around female bodily processes, these mischaracterisations also reveal a paucity of actual, thorough attention to the content of textual evidence connected to menstruation in the larger scholarly conversation. Just as we see the problem of medieval sources generalising the gynaecological problems and processes of women's bodies, we see a further overwriting and even exacerbation of this problem in contemporary scholarship. http://oldenglishthesaurus.arts.gla.ac.uk/category/?type=search&qsearch=menses&word=menses&page=1#id=1846 (accessed 9 January 2018).

41 Stein and Kim, *Flow*, p. 11. As they also note, 'It's actually a complex event, so much so that doctors and scientists don't fully understand it yet or what exactly it does … A big part of the problem is that, overwhelmingly, studies on menstruation tend to be funded by the "femcare" industry itself, and only, of course, to better develop and market their products' (pp. 12, 14).

42 An alternative spelling, *fleusa*, is exclusive to the *Vindicta salvatoris*, and refers to Christ's healing of the bleeding Veronica. See Swan, 'Remembering Veronica', p. 23. See also J. E. Cross, *Two Old English Apocrypha and Their Manuscript Source: The 'Gospel of Nichodemus' and 'The Avenging of the Saviour'*, Cambridge Studies

in Anglo-Saxon England 19 (Cambridge: Cambridge University Press, 1997), pp. 249–93. Christine Voth offers a brief but compelling reading of the Veronica tradition in 'Women and "Women's Medicine", Early Medieval England: from Text to Practice', in R. Trilling, R. Norris and R. Stephenson (eds), *Feminist Approaches to Anglo-Saxon Studies* (Amsterdam: Amsterdam University Press, 2023), pp. 279–316.

43 For a thorough treatment of the notion of wetness and fluids, see Conan Doyle, 'Anglo-Saxon Medicine and Disease: A Semantic Approach', 2 vols, PhD thesis (University of Cambridge, 2011), especially Chapter 5, 'Old English Physiological Vocabulary', where he discusses the strong affiliation of words for wetness with the concept of the humours, as on p. 22.

44 Sioban D. Harlow and Oona M. R. Campbell, 'Menstrual Dysfunction: A Missed Opportunity for Improving Reproductive Health in Developing Countries', *Reproductive Health Matters*, 8.15 (May 2000): 142–7 (p. 144).

45 Van Arsdall notes that Hubert DeVriend calls this 'common Ash', while Cockayne 'originally proposed that it was *Symphytum*. Bierbaumer does not positively identify this plant'; Anne Van Arsdall, *Medieval Herbal Remedies: The Old English Herbarium and Anglo-Saxon Medicine* (London: Routledge, 2002), p. 203 n. 230. The *Dictionary of Old English Plant Names* groups *ban-wyrt*, *galluc* and *hals-wyrt* under 'comfrey'; Peter Bierbaumer and Hans Sauer, with Helmut W. Klug and Ulrike Krischke (eds), *Dictionary of Old English Plant Names* (2007–09), http://oldenglish-plantnames.org (accessed 19 July 2023).

46 The passage reads: 'cnuca to swyþe smalon duste; syle drincan on wine. Sona se flewsa ætstandeþ' ('pound it into a fine powder; give it to drink in wine. The flow will stop quickly') (Niles and d'Aronco, *Anglo-Saxon Medical Texts*, Vol. I, p. 164 (60.1)); and 'gedrige hy ond cnuca to swiþe smalan duste; syle drincan on wine. Sona heo þa flewsan gewrið' ('dry it, and pound into a fine powder; give it to drink in wine. Quickly, the flow will be bound up') (p. 262 (128.1)).

47 Tiffany Beechy discusses the complex nature of binding, particularly with respect to language in the laws, charms and riddles. Of the charms, she suggests 'Their pragmatic function … is to "bind" elements of the real world in order to bring about some desired effect, such as a healthy birth or relief from a toothache', in *The Poetics of Old English* (Farnham: Ashgate, 2011), p. 85. Megan Cavell, in *Weaving Words and Binding Bodies: The Poetics of Human Experience in Old English Literature* (Toronto: University of Toronto Press, 2016), rigorously examines the conceptual metaphor of binding and weaving

in Old English poetics, thinking about woven objects, notions of bondage and constriction, and the woven-together nature of the body. Of the term *bindan*, she says 'when *bend/bindan/-sælan* and *searo* are invoked together there are two sets of connotations: that of hostile bondage, and that of cleverness and artistic skill' (p. 183). Even in the medical texts, which are not regularly poetic, the notion of binding or constricting menstruation functions in this same metaphorical register, alongside the literal.

48 Niles and D'Aronco, *Anglo-Saxon Medical Texts*, Vol. I, pp. 352 (178.6) and 346 (175.2). Van Arsdall notes the strangeness of Cockayne's choice to translate this whole passage into Latin, a sure indicator of his discomfort: 'His Latin translation and the supposed Latin original as given in DeVriend do not read the same. The Latin is talking about heavy menstruation' (Van Arsdall, *Medieval Herbal Remedies*, p. 225 n. 270). Further, the original Latin and Cockayne's different version suggest that Cockayne is not simply retreating to a Latin version, but has taken pains to retranslate the Old English version into Latin.

49 Van Arsdall, *Medieval Herbal Remedies*, p. 225 and n. 270.

50 Niles and D'Aronco, *Anglo-Saxon Medical Texts*, Vol. I, p. 346 (175.2). Van Arsdall translates this as 'It takes away all the smell of the fluid from her', whereas I read 'æþme heo gewrið' to indicate drying up/wrapping up by means of a vapour, particularly in relation to the similar remedy for nettle, with a lack of concern here with smell, and more with staunching bloodflow, although the two might well be related.

51 Ibid., Vol. I, p. 352 (178.6).

52 Cavell notes the use of *wriðan* in the context of medical remedies and metaphors, where metaphorical wounds are 'healed through a binding that parallels the wrapping of injuries'; Cavell, *Weaving Words*, p. 230. She notes the frequent use of the terms *bindan* and *wriðan* in the medical texts to indicate the binding and wrapping of wounds (p. 196 n. 7).

53 Cockayne, *Leechdoms*, pp. 331/333 (3.38.2).

54 Ibid., p. 330 (3.37.6).

55 Monica Green, *Making Women's Medicine Masculine: The Rise of Male Authority in Pre-Modern Gynaecology* (Oxford: Oxford University Press), p. 273.

56 *OEH* uses variations of the phrase *wið wifa monaðlican astyrigenne* (for the stirring of a woman's monthly cycle); Niles and D'Aronco, *Anglo-Saxon Medical Texts*, Vol. I, pp. 306 (150.1), 308 (152.1), 318 (158.2), 328 (164.1), 330 (165.4) and 342 (173.1).

57 The word *forstanden* appears only twice in the corpus, both in *LBIII* in reference to the same remedy. *DOE* defines this word, specific only to these occurrences, as meaning 'to stop, cease'.
58 Niles and D'Aronco, *Anglo-Saxon Medical Texts*, Vol. I, p. 328 (164.1).
59 Ibid., p. 318 (158.2).
60 *DOE*, 'forlætan', where 'to let, allow' is the first definition. This remedy is listed under definition 17, 'to leave off, cease, stop; break off, interrupt'. Most other remedies from the leechbooks appear under definition 19, 'to cease to contain, let escape, release (confined fluid); to let, shed (blood); release, discharge (bodily fluid acc.); 19.a. to unleash, let flow (bloodshed acc., upon the earth, to and dat.)'. These other remedies clearly invoke the flowing of blood, rather than restraining it, as the *DOE* suggests for three remedies, including 72.1 in *Bald*, and *OEH* 26.3.
61 *DOE* defines this use of the verb as 'to cleanse or purge of bodily impurity', and the use of *geclænsode* in the same remedy as to be 'purged of bodily impurity, of menstrual blood, or afterbirth'. As a comparison, a person may also be similarly 'cleansed' of demonic possession. Remedies for cleansing are discussed in Chapter 4.
62 *OEM*, in Niles and D'Aronco, *Anglo-Saxon Medical Texts*, Vol. I, p. 374 (2.3). This remedy also appears to be referenced in the chapter headings for *Bald*.
63 *DOE* defines both as 'flow of blood, bleeding, hemorrhage', with 'ryne' meaning 'running', and 'sihtan' meaning 'draining', in Bosworth–Toller. The desire for cleansing may well be motivated by patriarchal notions of cleanness, but a woman might also seek a different kind of cleansing. Voth also discusses remedies for abortion and stillbirth in 'Women and "Women's Medicine"'.
64 There is a specific category of remedy to help women purge or cleanse themselves of 'deadboren' or stillborn children, which I discuss in Chapter 4.
65 *OEH*, in Niles and D'Aronco, *Anglo-Saxon Medical Texts*, Vol. I, p. 330 (165.4).
66 Conception at this time was believed to be an extended process, culminating at forty days when the foetus was 'ensouled'. I discuss this at greater length in Chapter 4. Perhaps John Riddle refers to this remedy when he writes 'Anonymous recipe manuscripts written and copied at monastic scriptoria contain abortifacients (as menstrual regulators) and contraceptives. A ninth- or tenth-century manuscript has a prescription for cleaning the belly of a woman who cannot purge herself.' John M. Riddle, *Contraception and Abortion from the Ancient*

World to the Renaissance (Cambridge, MA: Harvard University Press, 1994), p. 104.

67 I do not suggest that the men using or writing this book fully understood or even recognised the potential of this remedy, although Green, 'Gendering Women's Healthcare', suggests that they may have. Rather, I suggest that it demonstrates the possibility of reproductive control for women, couched in language just vague enough and just uncomfortable enough to occlude its potential from those who might see it as abject.

68 *LBIII*, in Cockayne, *Leechdoms*, p. 330 (3.38.1). In its entirety: 'Wiþ þon þe wifum sie forstanden hira monaþgecynd wyl on ealað hleomoc and twa curmeallan sele drincan and beþe þæt wif on hatum baþe and drince þone drenc on þam baþe hafa þe ær geworht clam of beor dræstan and of grenre mucgwyrte and merce. and of berene melwe meng ealle to somne gehrer on pannan clæm on þæt gecynde lim and on þone cwið nioþoweardne þonne hio of þam baðe gæþ and drenc scenc fulne þæs ilcan scences wearmes and bewreoh þæt wif wel and læt beon swa beclæmed lange tide þæs dæges do swa tuwa swa þriwa swæþer þu scyle' (In case a woman's menstruation is obstructed: boil in beer brooklime and two centauries, give to drink, and bathe the woman in a hot bath, and drink the drink in the bath. Have already made for you a poultice of beer dregs and of green mugwort and celery and of barley flour, mix all together, stir in a pan, apply to the genitals and on the lower part of the vagina when she gets out of the bath, and drink a cupful of the same cup, warm, and wrap the woman up well, and let her be poulticed like that for a long time of the day. Do this twice or three times, whichever you must).

69 *LBIII*, in ibid., pp. 330/332 (3.38.2). Debby Banham and Christine Voth, in drafts of their forthcoming edition, translate it: 'You must always make the woman the bath and give her the drink at the same time, so that the nature/birth *æt ware ahsa* of it to the woman', indicating the difficulty of the passage that they are working to untangle (Debby Banham and Christine Voth (eds and trans), *Old English Medicine in British Library, Royal D. xvii*, Vol. II of *Anglo-Saxon Medical Texts*, Dumbarton Oaks Medieval Library (Cambridge, MA: Harvard University Press, forthcoming)). Stephen Pollington renders this last part thus: 'at the same time as would be normal for her [menstruation] ask this [time] of the woman', in *Leechcraft: Early English Charms, Plantlore, and Healing* (Ely: Anglo-Saxon Books, 2000), p. 394. Marijane Osborn notes, with reference to a different remedy, that 'only the emmenagogue brooklime would have the effect of expelling the placenta', suggesting its known efficacy for this function,

in 'Anglo-Saxon Ethnobotany: Women's Reproductive Medicine in *Leech Book III*', in Peter Dendl and Alaine Touwaide (eds), *Health and Healing from the Medieval Garden* (Woodbridge: Boydell, 2008), pp. 145–61 (p. 151).
70 Osborn, 'Anglo-Saxon Ethnobotany', p. 154.
71 Charlotte England, 'Erectile Dysfunction Studies Outnumber PMS Research by Five to One', *Independent* (19 August 2016), www.independent.co.uk/news/science/pms-erectile-dysfunction-studies-penis-problems-period-pre-menstrual-pains-science-disparity-a7198681.html (accessed 13 February 2020). Similarly, studies of coronary disease focus on men's symptoms and treatment, even in drug trials, which leads to significant adverse effects; Anita Holdcroft, 'Gender Bias in Research: How Does It Affect Evidence Based Medicine?', *Journal of the Royal Society of Medicine*, 100.1 (January 2007), 2–3, DOI: 10.1258/jrsm.100.1.2 (accessed 28 February 2020).

2

Fertility and pregnancy in the medical texts and prognostics

The Ishango bone, a dark, curved bone discovered in the Democratic Republic of the Congo, bears three columns of tally marks that suggest it might be a lunar calendar. This possibility prompted ethnomathematician Claudia Zaslavsky to write 'Now, who but a woman keeping track of her cycles would need a lunar calendar?'.[1] This observation sparked the interest of the internet many years later, which is how I found it, embedded in a meme and making the rounds on social media.[2] As the scholarly conversation around this object demonstrated, lunar calendars may be useful for other purposes, but, even so, this idea raises an important question about how women might have tracked their own menstruation in the time before personal calendars. The previous chapter focused on the importance of menstruation, either in addressing its absence, or its excessive presence, with one remedy noting that the physician should ask a woman the time of her regular cycle, which indicates, of course, that she knows that information: 'Þu scealt simle þam wife bæþ wyrcean and drenc sellan on þa ilcan tid. þe hire sio gecynd æt wære ahsa þæs æt þam wife' ('You must always make the bath and give the drink for the woman at the same time as her menstrual period might be. You must ask this time of the woman').[3] In this way, the remedies rely on women to be knowledgeable about their own internal rhythms; however, this kind of personal calendar must have been complicated for women who experienced nutritional disruptions and/or frequent pregnancy. In many ways, the counting of time works as both an internal and external measure of fertility and pregnancy; it is a measure that in contemporary America may be wielded as a weapon (as in abortion bans attached to a six-week gestational age), as well as a measure that in the Middle Ages would have relied on the knowledge and understanding of the pregnant person herself.[4]

Early medieval understandings of pregnancy derived from Aristotelian and Galenic models, which, though inaccurate, do link menstruation with conception and pregnancy. For Aristotle, conception takes place via the interaction between male semen and coagulated blood in the uterus after sexual intercourse, whereas for Galen, male and female semen combine together to make an embryo.[5] Neither Aristotle nor Galen correctly understood ovulation or fertilisation, though they recognised a relation among menstruation, sex and conception. Indeed, Lara Freidenfelds notes that researchers 'did not agree about the purpose of menstruation or the relationship of menstruation to ovulation until the 1930s', and that most authorities followed Hippocrates, who believed that 'women's bodies produced more blood than they were able to consume in their regular activities, so menstruation was necessary to rid the body of this excess blood', and that menstrual blood was 'retained during pregnancy in order to provide matter to form the fetus'.[6] Therefore, the tracking of menstruation was certainly a method of marking time in terms of pregnancy, even if the exact reasons for the lack of menses were not understood. And so, in this sense, external calendars – in whatever form that might have meant – would have been a means of tracking the internal calendar of a woman's menstruation and developing pregnancy.

The relation of time to pregnancy, even today, is vexed. Two very different notions of time are embedded in the pregnant body: time as measured by the world around the pregnant person, and time as measured inside the pregnant body. Of necessity, external time quantifies the internal rhythms of the body, and sometimes this external measure imposes rigid beliefs about what pregnancy should look like upon a body that does not abide by these expectations. Just as every woman's 'moon time' does not, in fact, cycle according to the phases of the moon, neither does every pregnancy follow the same schedule. Certainly, in both biological processes, certain phases of development occur in a specific order, but the limits of these phases are flexible and variable.

In addition to individual variation in timing, the contemporary method by which we measure pregnancy defies logic. In our contemporary system, a pregnancy begins the first day of a person's last menstrual cycle. That means that for most people, they are considered retroactively pregnant before they have conceived. This method, and ignorance around women's reproductive bodies, has led to no shortage of ridiculous political statements regarding pregnancy, wherein medical and scientific practices are seized on by often ignorant political figures in order to foment political opinion about abortion. For example, in 2012, Missouri's Republican Senate candidate, Todd Akin, publicly announced 'If it's a legitimate rape, the female body has ways to try to shut that whole thing down.'[7] Texas state representative Dan Flynn and Idaho state representative Vito Barbieri 'seem to believe the uterus can only be reached through an incision in the abdomen or via the digestive tract, respectively'.[8] Further, in 2019, Ohio lawmakers introduced (but did not pass) a bill 'that would have forced doctors to "reimplant" ectopic pregnancies – an impossible, fabricated procedure – or face criminal charges'.[9] Moreover, 'On the third day of his confirmation hearing to be a Supreme Court judge, nominee Brett Kavanaugh appeared to refer to birth control pills as "abortion-inducing drugs".'[10] Conflicts over the calculation of pregnancy, gestation and fertilisation rage in an era of increasingly precarious access to abortion. Outside the political misuse and misunderstanding of medical information, the standard method of calculating gestational age has its limits. Irregular menstruation, or even the cessation of menstruation due to breastfeeding or nutritional deficits, means that determining a 'last period' prior to pregnancy might not be accurate, or even possible.

If pregnancy in the twenty-first century is difficult to understand and quantify, particularly at the level of public discourse, medieval pregnancy cannot have been simpler. In fact, medieval understandings of conception used Aristotelian and Galenic principles, but also relied on pliable notions of timing: for instance, quickening.[11] At odds here are the documented or learned timelines of the Greek tradition, and the *felt* timelines of the pregnant person; in other words, there is a disjunction between when a person becomes pregnant actually, and when she realises that she is pregnant because she feels the movement of the foetus. The difference between these timelines is when learned men say a woman is pregnant, and when she says she is. The material in this chapter eddies around questions of time and knowledge, querying the differences between agency and influence attributed to women as they navigate fertility, conception and pregnancy. By placing medical texts in conversation with prognostic ones, I determine the ways in which these genres build alternative structures of time; where medical texts look forward and attribute agency to women, prognostics look backward, investing women only with ignorant influence over their pregnancies.

Prognostics by their very nature predict the future. While it is difficult to pin down a specific definition of prognostics that accurately blankets the genre as a whole, Roy Liuzza suggests that they 'differ from most later systems used to obtain knowledge of future events in the fact that they are calendrical rather than astrological'.[12] The early medieval English prognostics rely on timing and outcomes related to days, weeks and months, rather than relative to the positions of the stars in the sky. The relationship between medical and prognostic texts originates at least as early as Hippocrates, where prognostication was related to 'predicting the likely development of a medical condition. For Hippocrates and for the medical school founded by him, prognosis was the natural result of diagnosis, which looked at the signs and symptoms of a condition.'[13] Thus, while many medieval prognostics have little to do with medical prognoses, the genre has its origins in this ideology, and prognostics are often linked with medical remedies and charms in the scholarly tradition.

Even as prognostic texts predict the future, they do so from a retroactive position. In other words, a prognostic can only work as truthful from the position of a fulfilled prophecy, whereas a medical remedy offers women the means to assert their own will to achieve a desirable future for themselves. In this chapter, I first examine remedies for fertility that require women to take specific, concrete and knowing action in order to procure a desired future. Conception and fertility depend on exact timing, a kind of timing that would have been invisible and unknown to the bodies and authorities in question. Therefore, becoming pregnant is dependent upon the right combination of factors coming together in the right moment. Remedies for fertility call for the right actions to take place at the right times (and with the right people).

Alternatively, prognostics depict the pregnant person as a passive means of influence rather than agency, establishing the maternal body as a body to be read and interpreted by outside expert viewers. These texts actively revoke the agency of the maternal body, indicating instead the mother's passivity and ignorance. Following my discussion of the medical remedies for fertility and conception, I argue that the birth lunaria depict women as helpless to control the outcomes of their offspring, a kind of ineptitude and ignorance emphasised further in the embryological prognostic 'A Note on the Growth of the Fetus'. Where the birth lunaria offer a list of the lifetime outcomes for people depending on the day of their birth, 'A Note on the Growth of the Fetus' traces the timeline of foetal development, offering benchmarks for growth from the development of veins to the threshold for the possession of a soul. Despite the connection between quickening and ensoulment, discussed more fully in Chapter 4, 'A Note on the Growth of the Fetus' struggles to balance the reliance on maternal sensation to identify quickening with the emphasis on the mother's lack of awareness regarding the internal processes of foetal development until almost its very end.

Finally, I turn to the prognostic text 'The Omens in Pregnancy', which attempts to render legible the bodies of pregnant women in order to understand what precisely was happening inside them, and to predict future outcomes. These omens indicate that women have influence, but not agency, over the outcomes of their pregnancies, in stark contrast with the medical remedies. 'The Omens in Pregnancy' faults women for negative outcomes of pregnancy, using the signs of their pregnant bodies to predict outcomes ranging from sex to disability. These prognostics figure the (most commonly male) readers of the texts, who will also be the readers of women's bodies, as experts, while the women themselves remain ignorant and helpless. These prognostics offer a pretence of expertise and control over the pregnant body, but ultimately their attempts to render legible the ineffable body of the pregnant person rely on the existence of a future outcome to produce any meaning at all. In contrast, the knowledge and agency present in the medical texts allow women to respond proactively to their struggles with fertility and to become agents actively pursuing their own fertility goals.

Fertility and the conceiving body as contested territory

Women's actions and preferences are sharply delimited in many of the medical texts, which require them to remedy their own infertility, but which warn against the dangers of women's own agency. In writing about Carolingian infertility, Valerie Garver notes that 'Ecclesiastical and secular authorities believed women who were barren were often themselves at fault. This view accorded with the opinion that a wife ought to be chaste and honest', suggesting that infertility might be seen as a visible marker of a lack of piety, or worse, fidelity or chastity.[14] A woman of a higher social station who failed to conceive might well be fearful of the repercussions of her infertility.[15] The medical texts, so silent on ways of actually helping women give birth, however, offer a variety of methods for conception, most of which require a woman to take action to promote her own fertility, but carefully admonish her if she should threaten to overstep the limits of acceptable authority. Women seeking to conceive must bind items upon their bodies, drink concoctions that they must prepare, and participate in actions both medical and ritual in nature. The women seeking to conceive, unlike in most other remedies, are not only the recipients of action, but must take action themselves.

In some cases, fertility remedies require the direct intervention of the practitioner on the body of the woman, an action that is said to have immediate results. The *OEM* suggests that a knowledgeable practitioner must know the body of a deer in order to help the body of woman: 'Wið wifes geeacnunge: ban bið fonden on heortes heortan, hwilum on hrife, þæt ylce hyt gegearwað; gif ðu þæt ban on wifmannes earm ahehst, gewriðest scearplice, hræþe heo geeacnað' ('For a woman's conception: a bone may be found in the deer's heart, or sometimes in its womb, they have the same result; if you hang this bone on the woman's arm, bind it firmly, she will conceive right away').[16] The practitioner here must be so expert as to locate a bone inside the heart or reproductive organs of a deer, and to hang it ('ahehst') and bind it ('gewriðest') on a woman's body: she must be the passive recipient of action here, emphasising her role as the vessel waiting to be filled up by practices in which she cannot be expert.

However, remedies that require consumption of ingredients regularly require a woman to act and to participate actively in her own treatment. First, these remedies depend upon the woman's request for help to incite the action of the remedy. In the *OEM* remedy using a hare's testicle, the woman seems not to be the person preparing the drink, but she is certainly the person consuming it: 'haran sceallan wife æfter hyre clænsunge syle on wine drincan; þonne cenð heo wæpned cild' ('give the woman, after her cleansing, hare's testicle to drink in wine; then she will give birth to a male child').[17] The practitioner in this remedy is the enactor of only one explicit verb: he is to give, 'syle', the drink. Whereas the previous remedy indicates the many responsibilities of the expert, here the balance shifts, and while the practitioner probably also prepares the testicle in question, the remedy offers no specific requirements for the action. Instead, the remedy balances the action of the practitioner with the action of the woman. He gives, she drinks; ultimately, she gives birth – 'cenð' – to a child of the desired sex. Unclear, however, is the question of purging. Is this part of the purview of the expert, or of the woman? In either case, it is a prerequisite for this remedy to work, but no actor is named to the verb: the cleansing belongs to her, but we cannot tell who performs it. This body, however, is a demanding body. It is one that (a) requires cleansing (for a miscarriage? For menstrual concerns? For ritual purposes?), (b) seeks fecundity, and (c) desires a specific pregnancy outcome. This body wants something more; this body needs to prove a specific value, and acts in order to do so.

Like the prognostics, medical texts work to foreclose on the agency of maternal bodies through the implicit threat of damage to the child; remedies for the conception of male children rely on the expertise of men, at least, and often the active and knowing participation of male partners. Almost as a warning to a woman who would dare to undertake treatment for infertility without the knowledge and participation of her partner, this remedy from the OEM suggests that a woman who exceeds the limits of her femininity and encroaches upon the paradigm of masculinity will produce a child whose body reflects the dangerous blurring of the categories of gender. This remedy suggests:

> To þan þæt wif cenne wæpned cild: haran hrif gedryged and gesceafen oððe gegniden on drinc drincen butu; gif þæt wif ana hyt drinceþ, ðonne cenð heo androginem; ne byþ þæt to nahte, naþer ne wer ne wif.
>
> [So that a woman may give birth to a male child: let them both drink hare's womb, dried and scraped or crushed in a drink; if the woman alone drinks it, then she will give birth to an androgynous child, that is as nothing, neither man nor woman.][18]

Thus a woman has the ability to dictate the sex of her child – but also an injunction that to try to exercise such control independently would result in a literal transformation of her child's body. Indeed, this particular charm wants to remove the woman's own agency of growing a child: by leaving out the father, she risks giving birth to a child who is both male and female, not only thwarting the desired outcome of a male child, but also punishing her in a visible way for presuming a kind of mastery over the body clearly only meant for men, or at least not meant for women.

While the only remedy in the corpus for conceiving a girl also requires the active participation of both partners, it rigorously articulates the distinction between the sexes, emphasising the softness of women and the careful deployment of time necessary to conceive a girl. In fact, the intricate nature of timing and of the actions of the woman before, during and after sex emphasise her ability to dictate the outcomes of her conception. In its conflation of the woman with softness and even venery, it also figures her actions and consumption as crucially formative. Whereas remedies for the conception of a male heir are ubiquitous across cultures, rarely do medieval remedies offer advice for conceiving a girl. This remedy is one of the most elaborate, requiring two parties, actions before and after sex, consumption and application of medicines, and direction in other eating: one would almost think it might discourage parents from seeking a baby girl:

Wif to geeacnigenne: haran cyslybb feower penega gewæge syle on wine drincan þam wife of wife, and þam were of were. Ond þonne don hyra gemanan, ond æfter þon hy forhæbben. þonne hraþe geeacnað heo. Ond for mete heo sceal sume hwyle swamma brucan, ond for bæð smyrenysse. Wundorlice heo geeacnaþ.

[To conceive a female: give four pennies' weight of the dried stomach of a hare to drink in wine, the female's for the woman, the male's for the man. Then they should have sexual intercourse, and after this they should abstain. Then she will conceive right away. And for a while she should take mushrooms for food, and in the place of a bath, ointments. She will conceive wondrously.][19]

Like many other fertility and conception remedies in the *OEM*, this remedy calls for body parts from the hare, an animal associated with prolific fecundity. The onus of the consumption of the *wort* is shared, to a degree, between the would-be parents, dividing them into their expected sex roles. Thus, the remedy requires two different animals and two different brews, one using a male hare, and one a female, so that each party can conjure forth and assume the reproductive capacities of the specific animal, as they both drink: 'þam wife of wife, and þam were of were' ('the female's for the woman, the male's for the man'). In order to conceive a girl, it seems, there must be a balance between the two sexes that seems not to exist in other more general remedies for conception, or for the conception of boys. Perhaps this means that the seeking of a remedy for conception and the consumption of a remedy is associated with a kind of masculine proactiveness that is appropriate for (and perhaps even necessary for?) the conception of a son. Therefore, the remedy works to remind women of their female nature, thus also reminding them of their reliance on the male nature and action of their partners.[20]

While this remedy calls for both parties to consume the initial *wort*, the act of sexual intercourse is only the instigating moment of a longer timeline of conception. In other words: sex is only part of conception, and the postcoital actions of the woman have an effect on conception. After drinking their respective hare bits, having sex and thereafter abstaining, the remedy tells us 'þonne hraþe geeacnað heo' ('then she will quickly conceive'); however, intercourse is only the first part of the process of making sure the foetus is female. Therefore, although the remedy has created a space wherein both father and mother have responsibility for the getting of a child, it is ultimately the behaviours of the woman that dictate the final outcomes of its sex. Whereas 'The Omens in Pregnancy' suggest that the overconsumption of male-meats leads to a child with intellectual disability, here the remedy suggests she eat no meat at all, but rather only mushrooms: 'and for mete heo sceal sume hwyle swamma brucan' ('and for a while she should take mushrooms for food'). While 'for mete' is read by Niles and D'Aronco as the general 'as food', I would posit that the phrase suggests something more like 'in the place of meat', particularly as most dictionaries offer 'meat' as the first definition, followed by the more general possibility of 'food'.[21] The word *swamma* in fact is quite rare, occurring only five times in the corpus, and only once in the remedies.[22] As Neil Buttery suggests, 'Because mushrooms are notorious for their often narcotic and poisonous qualities, there [sic] were considered magic during the Middle Ages. Many an alchemist pored over the life cycle of fungi in an attempt to discover the secret of life itself – mushrooms had the amazing ability to create life from decay.'[23] Mushrooms do indeed spring up seemingly overnight, in unexpected and seemingly inhospitable and certainly abject places. Perhaps the dangers of mushrooms can account for their rarity in Old English, or perhaps it is their ineffable and magical potency: regardless, the instruction to replace meat with mushrooms *after* intercourse suggests that the conception of the foetus is still in process while the woman consumes the mushrooms, and her eating of them will be a deciding factor in the sex of the foetus that is conceived. Perhaps we might think of intercourse as the rain that falls on the ground, with the mushroom propagating as a result of this – the woman, then, is the spores of the mushroom, just waiting for something to spring up as a result.

Indeed, the second half of the remedy, to be undertaken after intercourse, focuses on calling forth the sexed qualities of the woman only. The woman is urged to forgo bathing in favour of an act synonymous with femininity: the smearing on of ointments: 'and for bæð smyrenysse' ('and in the place of a bath, ointments'). Just as mushrooms replace meat, so too do ointments replace bathing. This kind of bodily indulgence is also discussed in Homily Vercelli

VII, wherein women are figured as fundamentally flawed as a result of their 'softnesses'.[24] In response to a rhetorical question of why women are so 'sioce syn of hyra gecynde' ('sick from their condition'),[25] the answer negates the question of sickness but blames their *weakness* on the softness of their lifestyle:

> Ac hit <n>is swa: of hire liðan life hie bioð swa tyddre, for þan þe hie symle inne bioð 7 noht hefies ne wyrceaþ 7 hie oft baðieð 7 mid wyrtgemangum smyriað 7 symle on hnescum beddum hy r[e]stað
>
> [But it is <not> so: they are so weak on account of their soft lifestyle, because they are always inside, and they do not perform heavy work, and they bathe frequently, and smear themselves with unguents, and they always lie on soft beds.][26]

Here, the fundamental nature of women is softness and ease, and part of this ease is affiliated with excessive bathing (obviously prohibited in this remedy), but also explicitly with the 'smearing' of ointments.[27] Smearing often has affiliation with blessing and anointing, but that seems not to be the case either in Vercelli VII or in this remedy.

Vercelli continues to directly address the venial woman, uncoupling the notion of 'smearing' with 'health': 'Eawla, wif, to hwan wenest ðu þines lichoman hæle [geican] mid smyringe 7 oftþweake 7 oðrum liðnessum' ('Alas, woman, why did you expect to increase the health of your body with the smearing [of unguents], and frequent bathing, and other softnesses[?]').[28] Could this homily in fact be referring to the kind of practices we see in the *OEM*? Is the pleasurable smearing of Vercelli's woman the same as the smearing of the hopeful mother? Just two lines later, Vercelli associates the smearing, in fact, with lust: 'Gif ðu þonne his lustum symle fulgæst, þonne ne mæg he nawðer ne his mægen ne his fægernysse [gehealdan]' ('If you then follow [the body's] lust, then it may not keep either its strength nor its fairness').[29] Thus, women's practices of softness and leisure are markers of lust that the homilist claims weakens the body; in other words, smearing is not a remedy for health, because lust decays the body. However, this *OEM* remedy offers precisely the opposite: a woman is to consume fecundity itself in not one but two forms, and then, after sex, is to smear herself. Smearing of this sort is a feminine act, an act of leisure and womanly pleasure, and it is this specifically feminine act that is meant to help conceive not just any child, but specifically a female one.

This fertility remedy, one of the most involved and also perhaps one of the strangest, is full of contradictions, invoking a woman's fundamental venery and laziness while requiring her active agency. It suggests that she must be proactive but also demands her dependence on her partner. It suggests she should embrace her most feminine qualities and engage in scorned feminine practices, but also that she should be the instigator and organiser of the many parts of the remedy. This remedy pulls together the problems of female agency with the question of time, as well, in the way that time slips and exceeds the usual boundaries of conception. In order to place her at fault and require her responsibility, it grants her agency independent of her partner. While the strange lankiness of its vision of conception is visible in the postcoital and independent actions she must undertake, the disruption of the timeline is also visible in the opening and closing of the remedy. The end makes use of a word that is ubiquitous in medical and religious texts: *wundorlice*: 'wundorlice heo geeacnaþ' ('she will conceive wondrously'). Remedies across the board claim that they will work wondrously; indeed, this word occurs at least sixty times in medical texts. However, it occurs only thrice with reference to the healing of women: once as a way to stimulate menses, once to soothe sore nipples and here.[30] This remedy is the only one for conception that claims it will work wonderfully.[31] It frames this success as a future event: *geeacnaþ*, the present tense functioning as an implied future, situating the remedy itself in the moment of asking (please help me conceive a girl!), with the actions set in the future, to be undertaken later.

The remedy ends with kind of prediction of future success, but it also begins with an unusual verb form indicating continuing action: 'Wif to geeacnigenne' ('To conceive a female'). In my translation, I follow Niles and D'Aronco, who treat the verb as an infinitive in order to frame the sentiment of the remedy elegantly.[32] However, the verb here looks like a present participle, a form that is almost impossible to express without awkwardness in this particular context. For a woman to be conceiving? For the conceiving of a woman? Indeed, this form of this specific verb occurs only this one time in the entire corpus of Old English. There is something about time in this remedy: the remedy is in the future, but the conceiving that takes place in it reflects exactly this kind of progressiveness of the verb. It is not a perfect action, tidily completed, but rather one that is ongoing and whose limits are amorphous and difficult to encapsulate. It is about conceiving and not about conception. The remedy itself and the verbs it uses reflect the mysterious interior logic of the female reproductive body, and the way in which women's time and agency disrupt (push against, encroach upon) the rigid calendrical time and authority of the textual medical tradition at large.

Maternal ignorance in the Old English birth lunaria and 'A Note on the Growth of the Fetus'

Prognostics including the birth lunaria and 'A Note on the Growth of the Fetus' demonstrate a concern with the measurement of calendrical time relative to foetal development and birth, but ultimately these measures of time are used to demonstrate maternal ignorance rather than maternal agency. Whereas women struggling to become pregnant must be knowledgeable about their bodies and processes, pregnant women in the prognostics are completely subject to the time established by the nature of pregnancy itself. Their lives and the lives of their offspring depend entirely upon the accidents of their birthing calendars, and not upon anything they can do to dictate the timing of conception or birth. The birth lunarium included in MS Cotton Tiberius A.iii measures time in very specific and calendrical ways, codifying the helplessness of the pregnant person with regard to the vicissitudes of time and birth. Indeed, these prognostics are concerned with time in two segments: at the precipice between pregnancy and coterminous existence of foetus inside mother, and the future (often adult) life of the person being born. Similarly, MS Cotton Tiberius A.iii's 'A Note on the Growth of the Fetus' establishes an expertly known timeline of embryological development that indicates not the will, knowledge or agency of the mother, but rather her extended ignorance and reliance on the passing of time to reveal the truths of her birthing body.

The birth lunaria depend on the timing of birth to give meaning to a person's life. In erasing the mother from this equation, they set up the agency of the child and the timing of the child as almost independent from the birthing woman: in other words, they suggest that the child exits, not that the mother delivers. The template here is if/then: 'Gif man biþ accened on [ane] nihtne ealdne monan' ('If a man is born on a moon of one night old'), with days ranging from the one to thirty in the moon cycle.[33] The action is passive: the man is born. Even if the mother is invisible, she is an unnamed actor in the arrival and therefore in all future qualities of the person. The qualities posited span a person who will be sick, long-lived (three different days allow for this), 'in wordum leas' ('false in words'), fortunate (twice), martyred, a traveller, honourable, pious, useful, 'held in good esteem', a thief, destined to live a life of toil, frugal, a wastrel, 'neither poor nor rich' and friendly.[34] Only five of the prognostics focus upon the moment of birth and incipient time rather than on the distant future, each of these intimating a short life or difficult birth: 'se sweltað sona' ('he will die soon'), 'byð frecenlice accenned' ('be born perilously'), 'bið sona gefaren' ('soon be gone') and 'se bið sona gewiten' ('soon be departed').[35] While only one of these predictions is explicit about the danger of the birth, the rest imply an immediate, *sona*, death for children born on such days. Indeed, the prediction of the perilous birth is the only prognostic not to look beyond the moment of birth. It does not predict death, or characteristics in adulthood. It marks only as a singular characteristic the difficulty of the moment of birth – the sole shared defining quality of the children born on the ninth day of the new moon. While this birth lunarium is explicitly about birth, and not about pregnancy, it invokes automatically the question of time, and the calculation of pregnancy; the understandings of process of the development of the foetus; and the proper and, it seems, destined date of arrival.

While the work of most embryology differs from prognostics, 'A Note on the Growth of the Fetus' emphasises numerology and timing with respect to the parturient body, but, more importantly, to the embryo inside. This text peels back the occluding layers of the maternal body to delineate carefully the mysterious development of the foetus through time. Other early medieval embryologies appear in law codes, but this, the only extant Old English embryology, appears alongside clearly prognostic texts.[36] Rather than promoting medical or legal knowledge about foetal development, this text offers a numerological reading of the foetus, highlighting the natural order of its development almost completely divided from the maternal perspective and experience. Its reading of time indicates divisions among conception, quickening, ensoulment and the viability of the foetus to be born, with little attention to the knowledge and experience of the pregnant person.

The author attempts to make visible what is invisible inside the body of the pregnant person, sharing this knowledge with other (most commonly) male readers. In contrast to the knowing voice of the author, the pregnant person lacks control and understanding of what happens inside her, while the author figures himself as the expert. Offering one of the only explicit looks at a pregnant body in Old English literature, this text displays a month-by-month depiction of a pregnancy, which reveals as much about cultural attitudes to the pregnant body as about the foetus itself.[37] The titular line 'Her onginð secgan ymbe mannes gecynde hu he on his modor innoðe to men gewyrðeð' ('Here begins to tell about man's origin, how he becomes a man in his mother's womb') demonstrates this divide, indicating the primacy and action of the foetus, and the passivity of his mother, who serves only as a location.[38] She does not do the growing or nurturing, but rather he 'becomes', or even 'is made', which retains the passive structure removing action from the person doing the making.

The first trimester of pregnancy establishes the elements of the body, but the text makes clear that the foetus is not yet a person in the Christian sense. Despite the growth of a brain, covered by a membrane at six weeks; the development of a complex vein system, suggesting a heartbeat; and the division of the body into limbs, the foetus may possess a recognisably human body, but is not yet a person because, at the third month, still 'he biþ man butan sawle' ('he is a man without a soul').[39] The development of the brain at six weeks corresponds with the way the penitentials address the problem of abortion, wherein abortion after the forty-day mark is treated as murder, requiring a significantly more severe penance than termination of a pregnancy prior to this point. This is also the time before which the majority of miscarriages occur. This attitude toward personhood may have been necessary, or at least expedient, because of the high rate of 'spontaneous miscarriage ... where reproductive failures were not infrequent'.[40] Thus, this statement about personhood draws together concerns that are at once medical, spiritual and legal, demonstrating the difficulties of two persons inhabiting one body at a time when pregnancy was precarious and childbirth dangerous.

Just as the embryology reveals when the foetus does *not* have a soul, it similarly reveals maternal knowledge in a negative capacity. Even in the fifth month, wherein the foetus is supposed to have quickened, the mother remains 'witless', somehow unaware or ignorant of her pregnancy: 'On þam fiftan monþe he biþ cwicu. 7 weaxeð. 7 seo modur liþ witleas 7 þonne þa rib beoð geworden. Þonne gelimpð þæræmanigfeald sar þonne þæs byrþres lic on hire innoþe styrigende biþ' ('In the fifth month he is quickened, and grows, and the mother lies witless; and then the ribs are formed. Then she experiences much pain when the body of the fetus is stirring in her womb').[41] The word *witleas* means witless or senseless in its most literal sense and occurs forty-three times in the Old English corpus. It occurs in only one other place in the medical texts, where mandrake is used to treat insanity or possession.[42] Similarly, a small number glosses for *witleas* link it with ideas of dementia, torpor and devil sickness,[43] while the majority of other occurrences are in Ælfric's *Lives of the Saints* and homilies, where it consistently suggests ignorance and unknowing, often contrasted with coming to know things.[44] At worst, the passage seems to suggest complete ignorance on the part of the woman as to her state, indicating a firm disconnect between her body and her mind: the child has quickened and moves and grows, and yet this author seems to say the mother remains oblivious or insensate to the fact of her pregnancy, even as she is described as suffering pain specific to the movements of the foetus. An alternative reading, although it is not consistent with the general sense of this word, might mean the mother is uncertain about the outcomes of the pregnancy. In either case, or perhaps even in both at once, the *witleas* mother, even as she is halfway through her pregnancy, becomes *witodlice* – fully knowing or certain – only once she reaches the ninth month: 'On þam nigoþan monþe witodlice wifum bið cuð hwæder hi cennan magon' ('in the ninth month, it becomes known to the knowing woman whether they can give birth').[45] This passage emphasises the act of knowing, both in the verb and the adjective, actively reversing the structure of being without knowledge to knowing with certainty.

The mother in this description of birth is an ancillary figure. The text emphasises the foetus, and not the mother, turning her into a shadowy and ignorant figure, helpless against the changes in her body. Nothing in this passage serves to give comfort to an expecting mother as she conceives and experiences pregnancy; she is not the audience. In fact, she is not a part of the conversation about pregnancy; she is not even the subject. As the passage continues, little mention is made of the mother's experience as the child grows skin and bones in the sixth month; toes and fingers in the seventh month; organs, heart and blood in the eighth month. This description of the process of pregnancy and development of the foetus, attempting to provide a generalised, universal experience of the process, features a woman halfway through her pregnancy who is unaware of the quickened child growing inside her, but is simultaneously suffering multiple discomforts because of it. Such a description reveals an author completely disconnected from, or uninterested in, actual pregnant women, many of whom would be able to recognise their pregnancies not only by their lack of menses but by the movements of the quickened foetus. With respect to this text, these women are not the experts on their bodies; in fact, they know and understand almost nothing that is happening to them.

It is only just as she is about to be delivered of her baby that the hypothetical woman in this prognostic comes to realise what is happening to her body. The ninth month is marked by a woman's much-belated awareness of her conception and upcoming birth: 'On þam nigoþan monþe þitodlice þifum bið cuð hwaeþer hi cennan maʒon', which Cockayne translates as 'In the ninth month it is known to a woman whether she can bring forth'[46] Wilfrid Bonser as '… the woman knows for certain whether she may conceive',[47] and Liuzza as 'In the ninth month it becomes known to women whether they can give birth.'[48] These strange translations belie the difficulty of this passage; it simply does not make sense to insist that in most cases a woman would be unaware of her pregnancy until just before she gives birth, and of course this is not accurate. The word *cennan*, discussed at greater length in the following chapter, reveals the general trouble with Old English language around reproduction; it is non-specific at best and metaphorical at worst. The definition of *cennan* can stretch from 'beget' to 'conceive' to 'bring forth', therefore meaning anything from the moment of insemination to the moment of birth. In this particular context, the text offers two implications: (1) the woman is literally unaware that she has conceived a child until moments before she gives birth because she is so wildly dissociated from or ignorant of her own body; or (2) more optimistically, the woman is not secure in her ability to produce a living child until this final moment. While the latter is not impossible, given the fact of the extremely high maternal fatality rate, and in the context of the complicated word *cennan*, such optimism may be misplaced.[49]

This passage, and indeed this entire prognostic, serves to emphasise the mother's absence of control and awareness throughout the pregnancy, from conception to birth, focusing instead on the development of the child, independent of the witless state of the mother. Taken in its totality, the passage removes agency from the mother, and demonstrates her inability to participate in the continuation or outcomes of the pregnancy. Focused on the development of a foetus, this text writes out the woman's experience of childbirth, featuring her as merely a vehicle for her child, fundamentally detached from and uninvolved with the processes of development. Furthermore, her ignorance of her own pregnancy until very late means that she has little control over the continuation or outcomes of the pregnancy. This prognostic gives no description of birth – of what happens to the foetus during the process of birth or after birth. Instead, it suggests that the unborn foetus becomes toxic if it is not born before the tenth month, and, in true prognostic form, gives a day of the week upon which this is most likely to occur (Tuesday, in case you wondered): 'On þam teoþan monþe þæt wif hit ne gedigð hyre feore. Gif þæt bearn accenned ne biþ. Forþam þe hit in þam magan wyrð hire to feorhadle oftost on tiwesniht' ('In the tenth month, that woman will not escape with her life if the child is not born, because it will become a deadly malady in the stomach for her, most often on a Tuesday night').[50] The focus shifts from the developing foetus – unless we can count the transition from foetus to *feorhadl*, deadly malady – to the effect upon the mother. Upon failing to give birth in time, she cannot escape the disease of the unborn foetus. She is utterly subject to her pregnancy, and can exert no control over her body, but instead is dominated by it, and, in the end, can only submit to the requirements of her pregnancy, unable to do anything to protect, save or remedy herself.

The prognostics offer a frustrating access to Old English configurations of pregnancy and birth; the birth lunaria and embryology cannot exist without the birthing body, but the birthing body is not their concern. Rather, their focus on the foetus, and on the knowledge of outside viewers and speakers, contrasts explicitly with the ignorance of the pregnant person. The mother cannot control her pregnancy and decide when the baby will be born – she can only passively suffer the outcomes known by numerologists or the experts who have access to this textual tradition. She can die if the pregnancy goes on too long, but lacks insight into and understanding of the processes her body undergoes. These texts work to assert the knowledge of the expert, and to make clear that the woman herself knows almost nothing.

Pregnancy, influence and retroactive time in 'The Omens in Pregnancy'

Pregnancy is a time when the body manifests the passing of time in ways that are both readable and inexplicable. The contemporary pregnant body becomes a public object, making many pregnant women the targets of unwanted touching and advice; so too was the Old English pregnant body open to the reading of people outside that body. Like 'A Note on the Growth of the Fetus', the Old English 'Omens in Pregnancy' assert the authority and knowledge of outside viewers of the body, highlighting the lack of self-knowledge and awareness of the pregnant person.[51] These Old English prognostic texts use a range of physical cues to diagnose the internal state of a pregnancy. By their very nature, prognostic texts identify signs available in the material world to interpret and predict future outcomes. The prognostics for pregnancy look to the physical markers and behaviours of the pregnant person in order to interpret possible outcomes of the pregnancy. In doing so, they figure the reader of the text, who will also be the reader of the body, as expert, while they depict the pregnant person as ignorant and unknowing. These texts suggest that the pregnant body is legible, but only to external experts. Further, in demonstrating the consistent relationship between readable signs and future outcomes, the omens claim a reliable and systemic set of progressions of pregnancy. In doing so, they indicate that the outcomes of a pregnancy can be knowable based on the behaviours or body of the mother. While these omens ascribe authority and expertise to the readers of the pregnant body, they also indirectly assert the influence (although not knowing agency) of maternal preference and desire on the outcome of the pregnancy.

'The Omens' offer a series of six mechanisms by which such a viewer could interpret the body, ranging from a reading of her physical appearance (her eyes, the height of her belly), her physical mannerisms (how she walks) and her preferences (in flowers or food). What these characteristics reveal also varies, prognosticating anything from the sex of the child to its intelligence or physical shape. These prognostics seek not to warn women about the effects of their choices, but rather to render the mysterious pregnant body readable (presumably, to men), or to pinpoint women's behaviours as the causes of negative qualities in their children.[52] The qualities of the children at stake reinforce the function of unborn children as objects of value to be assessed by their possessors (their fathers and male relatives). Each of the characteristics correlates with elements of wergild-assessed value: whether the child will be a boy or a girl, whether the child will have physical or mental disabilities. In reading the pregnant body, the omens articulate a desire to predict and control future actions, locating the body in a knowable and predictable stream of time.

The omens that focus on the sex of the child are most concerned about the readability of the body, suggesting at once the ignorance of the woman who inhabits this body about its own conditions, and that an external expert can know it better than she does. Such a watcher can tell that 'gif heo gæð late 7 hæfþ hole Eagan heo cenneð cniht. Gif heo hraðe gæð 7 hafað aþundene eagan heo cenneð mæden cild' ('If she goes slowly and has hollow eyes, she will give birth to a boy. If she goes quickly and has swollen eyes, she will give birth to a girl').[53] A woman's pace as well as her physical appearance here relay information about her womb, suggesting that a woman is affected not only in terms of nutrition (the appearance of her eyes as either swollen or hollow), but also in terms of her physical capacity. The type of child she will bear literally changes the way she will walk, not just how she appears. Presumably the idea of slowness and hollowness with the male child suggests how much more work it is to grow a boy, with the girl seeming not to consume the woman's energy or fluids. Similarly, the third omen in this list suggests that 'gif þæt wif mid þam helum stæpeð' ('if she steps more with the heels'), she will bear a boy, as opposed to more 'mid þam tan' ('with the toes'), which indicates a girl.[54] The value of walking with the heels rather than the toes seems less about energy and wellness than a simple marker of difference, but again, it functions as a marker that is visible to all, but interpretable only by one who possesses this knowledge. The omen is not above relying on conventional wisdom regarding belly height (carrying high means a boy; 'gif hit byþ nyþer astigen heo cenneþ mæden' ('if it is hanging low she will give birth to a girl')), which at least focuses attention on the physical location of the foetus and how it sits in a woman's body.[55] Less about body and performance is the omen suggesting that a woman's preference for a lily over a rose indicates that 'he(o) cenð cnyht' ('she will give birth to a boy').[56] In this case, something intrinsic to the foetus exceeds the bounds of the womb and causes a woman to have specific preferences not for food, but for flowers, and it is only the savvy and educated observer who will know what this preference means. The woman acts only out of the necessity provoked by her pregnant state, having nothing to do with her own preferences or desires. The pregnant body is subject to the foetus, and readable by the men who watch her.

The final two omens in this set operate differently, and instead suggest that a woman's preferences are the cause of deficiencies in her child. Like the sex remedies, they indicate a kind of watcher who observes and interprets behaviour, although here it seems to be a diagnosis that occurs after that fact – when it is too late for a woman to change behaviour. Instead, these omens identify the source of the problem (in short: it is her). Perhaps unsurprisingly, the food preferences of a woman can have negative impacts on her child. The first omen suggests not only the dangers of specific preferences, but also the significance of timing, saying 'gif wif biþ bearneacen feower monoð oþþe fife 7 heo þonne gelome eteð hnyte oþþe æceran oþþe ænige niwe bleda þonne gelimpeð hit hwilum þurh þæt þæt þæt cild biþ dysig' ('if the woman is four or five months pregnant and frequently eats nuts or acorns or any fresh fruits, then it sometimes happens that because of that the child will be foolish').[57] This undesirable result derives from the coalescing of food craving and time: only under certain circumstances can the desire to eat nuts and fresh fruit lead to this outcome. The four-to-five-month mark in pregnancy indicates a specific kind of threshold; as the foetus quickens and becomes ensouled, it is also susceptible to the influences of maternal desires. Whereas the sex prognostics suggest that the woman's body reflects the qualities of the foetus through its appearance, action and preferences, instead here the foetus can be impacted by a woman's choices, and the impact is entirely negative, but also not entirely predictable. Instead, it is only *hwilum*, sometimes, that the eating of nuts and fruit in the fourth and fifth months can result in a child with mental deficiencies.[58] Given the indeterminate nature of this prognostic, there is no call for women generally *not* to eat nuts and fruit in these precarious months, but instead it is merely a diagnostic tool to be applied after the birth of the child, one designed not to advise but to admonish.

The final omen of this set similarly employs the structure of *hwilum* (sometimes) to point a finger of blame at women's behaviour. This omen suggests that:

> gef {heo} eteð fearres flæsc oððe rammes oþþe buccan oþþe bæres oþþe hanan oþþe ganran oþþe æniges þara neata. Þe strynan mæg þonne gelimpeð hit hwilum þurh þæt þæt þæt cild bið hoforode 7 healede.
>
> [if she eats the flesh of bulls or rams, or bucks or boars, or cocks or ganders, or of any animal that can engender, then it sometimes happens that because of that, the child will be hunchbacked and ruptured.][59]

Whereas the idea of nuts and fruit is more value-free, here the prognostic warns against the consumption of specifically male animals. These animals, the ones that can *strynan* – 'beget, generate, create' – are affiliated with the masculine principle of conception and fertility, as if eating the flesh of such a hypermasculine animal can cause these qualities to penetrate the porous pregnant body and make changes to the delicate foetus inside.[60] It seems to hint at the presumptuousness of a woman who might choose to eat such robust meat, hoping to take its masculine qualities into herself. The prognostic acts as a reminder not to exceed her female role; she is carrier and not engenderer. Perhaps even more than warning women, the prognostic works to reassure men that they are not the cause of birth defects in children, but rather that it is the hubris of women, those who are compelled to eat 'masculine' meat, that is to blame. The body of the pregnant woman – so fundamentally female in its work as carrier of the foetus – cannot help but be impacted by the force of masculinity should she try to consume it for herself. To attempt to exceed her role in such a way leads to a child who physically manifests this gender disorder through deformity, specifically becoming hunchbacked but, even more interesting, 'healede'. Liuzza translates this word as 'deformed', but what it means in specific medical terms is 'ruptured, suffering from hydrocele'.[61] Hydrocele is identified by swelling around the scrotum, usually in newborns, and is a 'fluid-filled sac around a testicle', which most frequently self-resolves.[62] One of the specific results of eating hypermasculine meat is damage to the masculinity of the foetus, however temporary such a malady might be. The desire of the mother to eat such foods seems beyond her control – it is an innate compulsion – but the omen reflects a fear of the presumption of a (reproductive) woman to exceed the boundaries of her sex. Such incursions into the arena of masculinity result in punishment via nature, and the social legibility of such punishment. Therefore, the prognostics depict pregnancy as a vulnerable time wherein the actions of a woman can indicate to an expert audience the goings-on inside her, but her actions can also provoke inward change, providing explanation (and blame) for disability in the child.

'The Omens in Pregnancy' rely on time and the consistent trajectory of pregnancy in order to read future outcomes or to explain past mistakes. They are invested in a particular moment – a moment when a pregnant body has not yet revealed its secrets. The results of actions or signs during pregnancy are only certified after the birth of the child, so the prognostic only matters in this interstitial moment.

It depends on the after but is only valid or important in the before. That so many of the omens rely on the construction of *hwilum* (sometimes) excuses but also unravels the certainty of prognostication. Suggesting that these signs or choices operate only 'sometimes' means that they cannot be proven false, but it also means that they demonstrate a lack of certainty. Despite the impulse of control and mastery over the unruly pregnant body, the fact that the outcome is only 'sometimes' predictable disrupts the authority of the prognostic. A system that claims women to be ignorant of their own bodies and preferences, but that also blames them for the outcomes of pregnancies, invests in women a great deal of influence over themselves and their offspring. That the prognostic can only occasionally identify the outcomes of a pregnancy undermines its reliability, a retroactive authority that was already precarious and that relied on after-the-fact pronouncements rather than in-the-moment protection.

Conclusions: Time and agency in treatments for infertility

The pregnant and conceiving body is one that operates on its own time but is also subject to the authority of expert physicians. The medical texts show us the difficult conflict in place for bodies that cannot conceive. Women are enjoined to seek the authority of experts and to include their partners, but they are also required to bear the responsibility for any perceived deficits in their progeny. If they cannot conceive, they are to blame, and thus it is incipient upon them to repair their fertility – but even then they cannot escape the authority of the textual, social and religious tradition. The message is: if there's a problem, it's your fault. You should try to solve that problem, but also you cannot because you are oblivious, or calculating, or exceeding the limits of your role as a woman. The problem is that the body is unreadable and uncooperative. It operates on its own schedule, so the textual tradition works to turn it into a text that can be understood and mastered.

Remedies for infertility vacillate between the notions that women can solve infertility on their own (with the help of medical experts) and that they must include their husbands. The final remedy I include here – a metrical fertility remedy from the *Lacnunga* quite long in its entirety – casts the net even wider, as a woman's fertility relies on her actions relative not only to those of her husband, but to her religious community as a whole. As she comes fully to occupy the role of a pregnant woman, rather than an infertile one, the agency she holds over her body is replaced by communal authority:

> Se wifman se hire cild afedan ne mæg: gange to gewitenes mannes birgenne ond stæppe þonne þriwa ofer þa byrgenne, ond cweþe þonne þriwa þas word:
>
> 'Þis to me bote, þære laþan lætbyrde;
>
> þis to me bote, þære swæran swærtbyrde,
>
> þis to me bote, þære laðan lambyrde'.
>
> Ond þonne þæt wif seo mid bearne ond heo to hyre hlaforde on reste ga, þonne cweþe heo:
>
> 'Up ic gonge, ofer þe stæppe, mid cwican cild, nalæs mid cwelendum, mid fulborenum, nalæs mid fægan.'
>
> Ond þonne seo modor gefele þæt þæt bearn si cwic, ga þonne to cyrican, ond þonne heo toforan þan weofude cume cweþe þonne:
>
> 'Criste, ic sæde, þis gecyþed.'
>
> [The woman who cannot carry to term her child: go to a dead man's grave and then step thrice over the grave, and then say these words thrice: 'This is my remedy for the loathed delayed birth. This is my remedy for the troubled dismal birth. This is my remedy for the loathed stalled birth.'
>
> And when that woman is with child and goes to her husband in bed, then she should say: 'Up I go, over you I step with a living child, not with a dying one, with a fully-gestated child, not with a doomed one.'
>
> And when the mother feels that the child is quickened, then she should go to church, and when she comes before the altar, she should say:
>
> 'To Christ, I have said, this is confirmed.'][63]

The remedy is structured in three parts: as the woman progresses from infertile to impregnated to quickened, her orientation to authority shifts. Even as she is the one to take action and to speak herself into potency, she is subject to the confirmation of those parties to whom she must make manifest her own body. The structure of *ond þonne* ('and then') sets up an explicit calendar of time relative to pregnancy, with quickening being the marker of a fully conceived foetus that can be announced not only to her partner but to the community at large.

While the woman is not explicitly faulted for actions she has or has not undertaken, as with deformities of the child listed in the prognostics, she is, in this situation, the primary party capable of responding to her state of childlessness. Her actions are twofold: physical movement and ritual declaration. She moves from the grave of a dead man to the bed of her husband to the church, expanding the circle of authority, culminating in a declaration to Christ before the altar. When she steps over the grave of the dead man, this action is lonely and isolated; this remedy imagines the desperation of a woman who cannot carry a child to term, who seeks a *bote*, a mending, a reparation, a restoration for three things: 'þære laþan lætbyrde ... þære swæran swærtbyrde ... þære laðan lambyrde' – in my own translation, 'for the loathed delayed birth, the troubled dismal birth, the loathed stalled birth'.[64] Each of these terms constitutes the only occurrence of the word in the Old English Corpus. This seems somehow both poetically appropriate and remarkable. The woman in this remedy seeks redress for a problem that is at once universal and heartbreakingly unique to her. This is not a woman who cannot conceive. She is a woman who cannot give birth to a healthy child. The problem is entirely hers, as she suffers through miscarriage and seeks remedy at the grave of a dead man (and specifically a man). Only when she is pregnant does she find company: the body she steps over belongs to her partner. But they have experienced this moment before, the remedy implies. It is not until the foetus has quickened that the confirmation of her pregnancy by the authority of the church is appropriate. Lisa Weston notes the power implicit in the woman's incantation and increasingly public performance, from dead man to living man to entire church community, ultimately suggesting that 'Through her charm the mother has bespoken herself potent and fertile; her words have made her womb a site of transformation, of the nonliving becoming living, the inchoate taking form.'[65] It is through her actions, and more importantly through her voice, that the woman can speak a foetus into being.

And it is this that tells us what it is to be pregnant at this time: to be profoundly alone, but also to be an object to be read, that must speak itself, but then be spoken over. The woman in this remedy is a far stretch from a woman who has no idea she is about to give birth until the very month she will do so. Here the woman must recognise the problem, seek out a solution and carry out that solution, in part independently, and in part with the help of her community. She must recognise when she becomes pregnant so that she can safeguard that pregnancy by announcing it publicly, both confirming and protecting it by doing so within the confines of the church. But if she has power, she also has responsibility, and the burden is upon her to produce a child who will ultimately become the property of her husband.

It is moments like this that lead Weston to argue that sections of the leechbooks that are devoted to women exclusively 'evoke a female oral tradition existing along-side of and in dialogue with the dominant male traditions'.[66] We may read infertility remedies like this one as practices that place women in a position of authority and agency over their bodies in a way that many of the other responses to pregnancy in the leechbooks do not. Such a reading is certainly plausible, although we must not neglect the implications of the moments in which women are declined agency (determining and controlling the positive qualities of the developing foetus), and the ones in which they are offered it (contributing to disabilities and responding to infertility). Such an implicit critique of women's control over their own (faulty) bodies seems entirely consistent with a tradition that denies women's understanding of the very nature of their own reproductive bodies.

The remedies for fertility and prognostics for pregnancy taken together create a picture of pregnancy drawn and interpreted by men who saw themselves as authorities on the bodies of women, but who also had little skill or ability to dictate any real control over these bodies. The desire to impose limits seems a way of imposing order on something resistant to external structurality. Women evade and yet appear in these texts, depicted by male authorities. As in the prognostics, they function as objects to be read and interpreted by those who know better, know more. And yet they retain a kind of agency that escapes the limits of legibility, and that reveals more about medical ignorance and impotence than about masculine authority.

Notes

1 Claudia Zaslavsky, 'Women as the First Mathematicians', *Newsletter of the International Study Group of Ethnomathematics*, 7.1 (1992), 1.
2 For a solid discussion of the origins and internet presence of this meme, see Veritas-Certum, 'The Ishango Bone: A 22,000-Year-Old Lunar Calendar Made by Women as the First Mathematicians', www.reddit.com/r/badhistory/comments/m5hzjw/the_ishango_bone_a_22000_year_old_lunar_calendar/ (accessed 6 July 2023).
3 Thomas Oswald Cockayne, *Leechdoms, wortcunning, and starcraft of early England. Being a collection of documents, for the most part never before printed, illustrating the history of science in this country before the Norman Conquest*, 3 vols (London: Longman, Green, Longman, Roberts and Green, 1864–66), p. 330 (38.1).
4 In June 2022, the United States Supreme Court overturned *Roe vs Wade*, which resulted in significant limits to access to abortion. For context, please see David S. Cohen, Greer Donley and Rachel Rebouché, 'The New Abortion Battleground', *Columbia Law Review*, 123.1 (January 2023), 1–100. See also Kaiser Family Foundation (KFF), 'Abortion in the United States' (1 July 2022), www.kff.org/womens-health-policy/press-release/abortion-in-the-united-states/ (accessed 15 July 2023).
5 Alex Lopata explains that 'Aristotle proposed that in mammals, including humans, an egg was formed in the uterine cavity and conception occurred by the action of the male semen on coagulated blood in the uterus, soon after mating. Galen (129–210 ACE) taught that the semen of women originated in the female testes and travelled via the fallopian tubes to the uterus, where it mingled with the male semen to produce an embryo … The ideas of these two teachers persisted for over a thousand years … [and not until William Harvey (1598–1601)] did anyone question where and how the egg and embryo are formed.' Alex Lopata, 'History of the Egg in Embryology', *Journal of Mammalian Ova Research*, 26.1 (2009), 2–9 (p. 2).

6 Lara Freidenfelds, *The Modern Period: Menstruation in Twentieth-Century America* (Baltimore: Johns Hopkins University Press, 2009), pp. 45, 24.
7 Sean Sullivan, 'Todd Akin Takes Back Apology for "Legitimate Rape" Comment', *Washington Post* (10 July 2014), www.washingtonpost.com/news/post-politics/wp/2014/07/10/todd-akin-takes-back-apology-for-legitimate-rape-comment/ (accessed 6 July 2023). In this piece, Sullivan offers context for the original 2012 statement, the television commercial apology and the book, wherein he retracts the apology and claims that his original statement was misinterpreted. For media treatment of the story after the initial comment, see David Cohen, 'Earlier. Akin: "Legitimate Rape" Rarely Leads to Pregnancy', *Politico* (19 August 2012), www.politico.com/story/2012/08/akin-legitimate-rape-victims-dont-get-pregnant-079864 (accessed 24 June 2022).
8 Christina Cauterucci, 'Ignorance Is Blessed', *Slate* (15 May 2019), https://slate.com/news-and-politics/2019/05/alabama-abortion-law-republican-ignorance-female-reproduction.html (accessed 3 March 2020). See also Jill Filipovic, 'Alabama's Abortion Bill Is Immoral, Inhumane, and Wildly Inconsistent', *Vanity Fair* (15 May 2019), www.vanityfair.com/style/2019/05/alabamas-abortion-bill-is-immoral-inhumane-and-wildly-inconsistent (accessed 6 July 2023); and Bill Barrow, 'Alabama Governor Invokes God in Banning Nearly All Abortions', AP News (16 May 2019), https://apnews.com/article/7a47ddc761dc4b72a017b0836da3a87b (accessed 6 July 2023).
9 Nida Allam, 'Ectopic Pregnancies Are Medical Emergencies – Not Political Footballs', *Teen Vogue* (1 April 2022), www.teenvogue.com/story/ectopic-pregnancy-abortion (accessed 24 June 2022). See also Timothy Williams, 'New Abortion Bills Are So Tough that Some Conservatives Have Qualms', *New York Times* (4 December 2019), www.nytimes.com/2019/12/04/us/abortion-bills-ohio-ectopic-pregnancy.html (accessed 6 July 2023).
10 Anna Almendrala, 'Why Do Conservatives Still Think Contraception Is Abortion?', *Huffpost Health* (7 September 2018), www.huffpost.com/entry/conservatives-contraception-abortion_n_5b92fd41e4b0cf7b003fc28a (accessed 3 March 2020). See also Ariane de Vogue and Veronica Stracqualursi, 'Kavanaugh "Abortion-Inducing Drug" Comment Draws Scrutiny', CNN (7 September 2018), www.cnn.com/2018/09/07/politics/brett-kavanaugh-hearing-birth-control/index.html (accessed 6 July 2023).
11 John Riddle suggests, based on the thirteenth-century treatise *Women's Secrets*, that there was a 'common understanding among women. They

believed that there was an interval between the deposit of a man's semen and the uncertain point at which a woman's body turned the man's seed into an embryo. Latin terms for what we call an embryo were *conceptus*, *embryo*, and *fetus*. In modern speech we distinguish between an embryo, which we define as the first three months of a fertilised egg, and a fetus, a child *in utero* after three months of development. Neither the Middle Ages nor the classical antiquity of the Romans and Greeks made such distinctions.' John M. Riddle, 'Contraception and Early Abortion in the Middle Ages', in Vern L. Bullough and James A. Brundage (eds), *Handbook of Medieval Sexuality* (New York: Garland, 1996), pp. 261–77 (p. 264).

12 R. M. Liuzza, *Anglo-Saxon Prognostics: An Edition and Translation of Texts from London, British Library, MS Cotton Tiberius A.iii* (London: D. S. Brewer, 2011), pp. 1–2. L. S. Chardonnens critiques the definitions stated in Philip Pulsiano and Elaine Treharne (eds), *A Companion to Anglo-Saxon Literature* (London: Blackwell, 2017), noting 'First, prognostication does not necessarily deal with "bad fates or unfortunate outcomes". Therefore, prognostics do not so much warn as inform their users. Second, there can be no question of a "probable occurrence of events", because prognostication does not allow for probability: it offers certainty. Third, it is true that most prognostic genres are temporal, i.e. structured by time sequences, but there are also genres which are non-temporal, e.g. alphabetical dream books.' L. S. Chardonnens, *Anglo-Saxon Prognostics, 900–1100* (Leiden: Brill, 2007), p. 6. I disagree only with the claim that prognostics are certain, as I will include evidence of prognostics that include 'possible' outcomes, or outcomes that only happen 'sometimes'.

13 British Library, description of Hippocrates, *Prognosticon*, https://www.bl.uk/collection-items/historiated-initial-of-a-doctor-teaching-urine-examination-to-students-from-hippocrates-prognosticon (accessed 24 June 2022).

14 Valerie Garver, 'Childbearing and Infancy in the Carolingian World', *Journal of the History of Sexuality*, 21.2 (May 2012), 208–44 (p. 220). Garver further suggests that 'Ecclesiastical writings such as these promoted religious solutions to the problem of infertility. That few individuals probably knew anything about biological reasons for infertility other than aging or much about safe gynecological and obstetrical practices underlines the importance of prayers for fertility performed by the Carolingian elite' (p. 221), but also notes that men were occasionally seen as responsible for infertility: 'In his *De institutione laicali* (Concerning the institution of the laity) of the 820s, Jonas of Orléans

wrote that men who wasted their seed by having sex with their pregnant wives might turn their fecundity to sterility. Citing Augustine of Hippo, he added that the sinful acts of married men could cause impotence. Men, it seems, could also be blamed for the inability of a couple to have children, though the repercussions for women accused of the same problem were far worse than the shame or anxiety a childless husband might endure for lack of a male heir' (p. 221).

15 Edith, wife of Edward the Confessor, for example, went to great pains to assert the chastity of their marriage, a significant part of the claims for his canonisation. However, according to Susan Abernathy, 'Modern historians are now proponents that they did have sex and just didn't have any children. This barrenness in marriage was to have a forceful and direct impact on the history of England'. Susan Abernathy, 'Edith of Wessex, Queen of England', www.medievalists.net/2013/02/edith-of-wessex-queen-of-england/ (accessed 27 June 2022). See also Pauline Stafford, *Queen Emma and Queen Edith: Queenship and Women's Power in Eleventh-Century England* (Hoboken, NJ: Wiley Blackwell, 2001).

16 John P. Niles and Maria D'Aronco (eds and trans), *Anglo-Saxon Medical Texts*, Vol. I, *The Old English Herbal, Lacnunga, and Other Texts*, Dumbarton Oaks Medieval Library (Cambridge, MA: Harvard University Press, 2023), p. 380 (3.17).

17 Ibid., p. 388 (5.13).

18 Ibid., p. 386 (5.12).

19 Ibid., p. 388 (5.14).

20 A remedy for the conception of a girl or a boy specifically is not necessarily a remedy for infertility, although of course it could be. However, the fact that such a remedy calls for action on the part of both parties opens the door to speculation that infertility might also be caused by either or both parties. In seeking to remedy something in not just the woman, but also in the man, it suggests a need for treatment that could place the fault in either body.

21 Niles and D'Aronco, *Anglo-Saxon Medical Texts*, Vol. I, p. 389. Both Bosworth–Toller and Clark Hall suggest the definition as 'meat. Food'; J. R. Clark Hall, *A Concise Anglo-Saxon Dictionary*, 4th edn (Cambridge: Cambridge University Press, 1960), p. 234; and Joseph Bosworth, 'METE', in *An Anglo-Saxon Dictionary Online*, ed. Thomas Northcote Toller, Christ Sean and Ondřej Tichy (Prague: Faculty of Arts, Charles University, 2014), https://bosworthtoller.com/22712 (accessed 23 December 2023). Kathryn Maude argues that *brucan* is Ælfric's word for forbidding sex during Lent, in the context of enjoying meat rather than enjoying a woman, in *Catholic Homilies* I, 11.

This word therefore takes on a venial and sexualised connotation; Kathryn Maude, *Addressing Women in Early Medieval Religious Texts* (Woodbridge: Boydell and Brewer, 2021), p. 27. Notably, Sally Crawford suggests that the ubiquity of intestinal parasites may well have made this mushroom remedy dangerous for women: 'intestinal parasites – roundworm, whipworm and tapeworm – were a commonplace, and vitamin and iron deficiencies would have been chronic, especially for women. Under these circumstances, the remedy for infertility that recommended replacing meat with mushrooms in the diet would have been positively harmful if followed.' Sally Crawford, *Childhood in Anglo-Saxon England* (Stroud: Sutton, 1999), p. 58.

22 According to a search of the *DOE Web Corpus*, three of the occurrences are glosses, and the only other fuller use of the word is in the *Peri Didaxeon*, wherein the mushroom is to be salted; Antoinette diPaolo Healey, with John Price Wilkin and Xin Xiang (eds), *Dictionary of Old English Web Corpus* (Toronto: Dictionary of Old English Project, 2009). Jane Roberts, Christian Kay and Lynne Grundy, *A Thesaurus of Old English* (Leiden: Brill, 2000), offer only *swamma* (with variations in prefix: *feldswam* (toadstool), *meteswam* (edible mushroom)) as the word for fungus/mushroom. Despite the certain ubiquity of this ingredient, it seems quite odd that there are so few occurrences, and, especially, that no other remedies make use of it. https://oldenglishthesaurus.arts.gla.ac.uk/category/?type=search&qsearch=mushroom&word=mushroom&page=1#id=3227 (accessed 28 March 2020).

23 Neil Buttery, 'On a Mushroom Hunt', *British Food: A History* (6 November, 2012), https://britishfoodhistory.com/2012/11/06/on-the-hunt-for-mushrooms/ (accessed 28 March 2020). John Marco Allegro, in *The Sacred Mushroom and the Cross* (London: Hodder and Stoughton, 1970), believed the *Amanita muscaria* mushroom was a religious fertility sacrament, although, as Richard J. Miller notes in 'Religion as a Product of Psychotropic Drug Use', *The Atlantic* (27 December 2013), Allegro's hypotheses 'were not well received. Many Christians took exception to the fact that he believed that Jesus never existed and was really just a code word for a giant phallus-shaped magic mushroom.' In Celtic tradition, mushrooms are often associated with fairies, potentially because of the psychedelic properties of two types of Irish mushroom. See 'The Mysterious and Lost Magic Mushroom Rituals of the Ancient Celts', in *The Genuinely Irish Old Moore's Almanac*, https://oldmooresalmanac.com/the-mysterious-and-lost-magic-mushroom-rituals-of-the-ancient-celts/# (accessed 28 March 2020).

24 Samantha Zacher, 'The Source of Vercelli VII: An Address to Women', in Samantha Zacher and Andy Orchard (eds), *New Readings in the Vercelli Book* (Toronto: University of Toronto Press, 2009), pp. 98–149. Translations of this source are hers. Kathryn Maude notes: 'Similarly, Vercelli VII, a tenth-century Old English homily translated from a sixth-century Latin sermon, is assumed to have been written for a mixed audience based on its inclusion of an address to women. Women are only included in Vercelli VII when addressed directly, however, and are not included in its address to the generic Christian listener.' Maude, *Addressing Women*, p. 172.
25 Zacher, 'Source of Vercelli VII', p. 137, lines 56–7.
26 Ibid., p. 137, lines 57–9.
27 A common term, it occurs hundreds of times in various forms, but typically refers to ceremonial anointing, for example the biblical washing of feet and anointing with oils such as myrrh. In the form *smyre*, as in the verb 'to smear', it occurs frequently in the medical texts, but in this particular form, to have a 'smearing', it occurs in only this remedy, according to the *DOE Web Corpus*.
28 Zacher, 'Source of Vercellin VII', p. 140, lines 73–4.
29 Ibid., p. 140, lines 76–8.
30 See *OEH* 19.3 and 152.1. In contrast, it occurs far more regularly among other remedies: thirty-three times in the *OEH*, twenty-two in *OEM* and five in *Bald*.
31 *OEM* 3.17 uses a similar formula, but claims she will conceive *hræþe*, quickly, rather than wonderfully. The notion of a quick conception is equally compelling: does it suggest she will only need to perform the remedy once, and thus it is quick? Or does it speed up the pace of conception, which here in this remedy seems to be somewhat leisurely?
32 Niles and D'Aronco, *Anglo-Saxon Medical Texts*, Vol. I, p. 389.
33 Liuzza, *Anglo-Saxon Prognostics*, p. 202.
34 Ibid., pp. 202.4.
35 Ibid., pp. 202.5, 202.8, 202.9, 202.15, 202.20, 202.17.
36 I follow Liuzza, who argues that while this embryology shares much with other European embryologies, it lacks an immediate source. Liuzza argues against Chardonnens, who suggests that this prognostic is a version of Vindicianus: 'The text is found only here; it has been little studied and its sources are not known. Chardonnens points out that analogous texts in Old Frisian and Old Saxon are found not in medical collections but in law codes, where they help define the legal status of a pregnant woman and her unborn child. He argues that the text is a version of Vindicianus's *Gynaecia*, c. 21 (on the fetus) but this is a seriously misleading characterization. The fourth-century Gynaecia

survives in a number of very different versions, but none of them is remotely like T14 ['Note on the Growth of the Fetus'] ... T14 bears some similarities to a brief anonymous text on this subject in Paris, BNF, nouv. Acq. Lat. 1616m 12r: notable parallels include the formation of the brain in the first month ... and the quickening of the fetus in the fifth month. T14 is most closely similar, however to a text in Leiden University Library, Vossianus lat. Q.69, 26v; in fact it is largely a translation of the Leiden text (though the last sentence in T14 does not appear in the Latin). Contrary to Chardonnens's assertion, however, the Leiden text is not an excerpt of Vindicianus – it has no verbal parallels to any version of Vindicianus printed in Rose or noted by Cilliers, and its indications for the various months are quite different from those found in published versions of Vindicianus's texts.' Ibid., p. 58.

37 Zubin Mistry argues that many embryologies provide symbolic information relative to Christian ideologies rather than contemporary medical knowledge: 'Most embryological texts in circulation were not, strictly speaking, medical embryologies. They elaborated numerological or allegorical readings of fetal development; the fetus was the means to other intellectual ends ... The pervasions of evocations and symbolic representations of the fetus in early medieval culture is no surprise. The central moment in Christian theology, Christ's incarnation, began in Mary's womb.' Zubin Mistry, *Abortion in the Early Middle Ages, c. 500–900* (Woodbridge: Boydell and Brewer, 2017), p. 15. This embryology seems more inclined to the medical than the Christological, as it focuses on physiological developments as well as ensoulment.

38 Liuzza, *Anglo-Saxon Prognostics*, p. 200.

39 Ibid., p. 200.4.

40 Mistry, *Abortion*, p. 141.

41 Ibid., p. 200.4.

42 Bosworth–Toller, 'wit-leás': 'Wið gewitleaste, þæt is wið deofulseocnysse, genim of þam lichoman þysse ylcan wyrte mandragore þreora penega gewihte, syle drincan on wearmum wætere swa he eaðelicost mæg' (For insanity, that is, against devil-sickness, take from the body of the mandrake plant three pennies' weight, and give to drink in warm water so that he will be easily cured). Bosworth, *An Anglo-Saxon Dictionary Online*, 132.4.

43 See *DOE Web Corpus*.

44 For example, in Ælfric's 'Life of St Thomas', where the queen of King Mazdai is asked to reason with Migdonia, but she reports back that Migdonia has not in fact lost her wits: 'Heo cwæð eft him to, Ge cwædon þæt min swuster, and ic sylf eac wende, þæt heo gewitleas

wære; ac heo soþlice becom to soþum wisdome on þam heo me dyde dælnimend þæs ecan lifes' ('Ye said that my sister – and I myself likewise thought so – was witless; but she hath verily come to true wisdom'); Ælfric, *Ælfric's Lives of Saints*, ed. W. W. Skeat, trans. Miss Gunning and Miss Wilkinson, 2 vols, Early English Text Society, o.s. 114 (London: Kegan, Paul, Trench, Trübner, 1900), pp. 413–15.
45 Ibid., p. 200.4.
46 Cockayne, *Leechdoms*, p. 146.
47 Wilfrid Bonser, *The Medical Background of Anglo-Saxon England* (London: Publications of the Wellcome Historical Library, 1963), p. 265.
48 Liuzza, *Anglo-Saxon Prognostics*, p. 201.
49 Duncan Sayer and Sam D. Dickinson, 'Reconsidering Obstetric Death and Female Fertility in Anglo-Saxon England', *World Archaeology*, 45.2 (2013), 285–97 (p. 293).
50 Liuzza, *Anglo-Saxon Prognostics*, p. 200.
51 'The Omens' are found in London, BL, MS Cotton Tiberius A.iii, a manuscript associated with prognostic texts. See ibid.
52 While often these kinds of predictions are the purview of women's conversation, their existence in a text suggests a likely male audience, or at least an audience of people who will never give birth. Laywomen's literacy was significantly limited at this time, and so while religious women might have had access to literacy and texts like this one, their relations with such texts most probably would have been as textually informed experts, not as purveyors or seekers of personal experience.
53 Liuzza, *Anglo-Saxon Prognostics*, p. 212.
54 Ibid.
55 Ibid. Interestingly, this correlation of high to a boy and low to a girl is counter to modern interpretation, which seems to suggest that a high belly is correlated with a female foetus. Janey Adams, 'Old Wives' Tales, Debunked', NPR (2 August 2011), www.npr.org/sections/babyproject/2011/08/02/138549731/old-wives-tales-debunked (accessed 3 March 2020).
56 Liuzza, *Anglo-Saxon Prognostics*, p. 212.
57 Ibid.
58 *Dysig* appears 232 times in the *DOE Web Corpus*, often in an adjectival function. It is difficult to be certain about the seriousness of the term – whether it means simply 'foolish' in the prognostic context, or whether, given the vaguely medical nature of the genre, it suggests a more serious kind of intellectual disability. The term occurs most frequently in explicitly religious contexts, as in Ælfric (twenty-nine occurrences) and Alfred's translation of Boethius (thirty occurrences).

It does not appear to occur in lawcodes, and only occurs once elsewhere in the medical genre, in the heading of *Bald*, where a group of remedies seek to treat 'ungemynde and wiþ dysigum' (dementedness/insanity and foolishness); Cockayne, *Leechdoms*, Vol. II, p. 142 (66.1). I suspect that in this kind of medical context *dysig* is understood not just as a kind of ordinary foolishness, as elsewhere in the corpus, but rather as a more fundamental kind of disorder, such as mental illness.

59 Liuzza, *Anglo-Saxon Prognostics*, p. 212.
60 Bosworth, 'strynan', in *An Anglo-Saxon Dictionary Online*.
61 Liuzza, *Anglo-Saxon Prognostics*, p. 213. DOE, 'healede'. Interestingly, this word also occurs twice in the *Herbarium*, and fewer than ten times in the corpus altogether, most frequently glosses.
62 Mayo Clinic, 'Hydrocele' (updated 12 January, 2023), www.mayoclinic.org/diseases-conditions/hydrocele/symptoms-causes/syc-20363969 (accessed 8 July 2023).
63 Niles and D'Aronco, *Anglo-Saxon Medical Texts*, Vol. I, pp. 510/512 (161).
64 Niles and D'Aronco translate these phrases as 'hateful delayed birth ... grievous black birth ... hateful lame birth' (ibid., p. 513). I agree with their understanding of 'lætbyrde' as 'delayed birth', probably a labour that stalls or takes too long, thus resulting in the death of the foetus. They treat 'swærtbyrde' (black birth) in a way that takes the adjective literally; I prefer to translate it as 'dismal', removing colour markers from negative experiences. 'Lambyrde' offers a challenge, particularly in contemporary language for disability; Bosworth–Toller defines the phrase as 'a lame, weak, imperfect birth', while Clark Hall defines *lama* as 'crippled, "lame", paralytic, weak' (*Concise Anglo-Saxon Dictionary*, p. 210). The notion of a birth as 'lame' in the literal sense is perplexing – a birth cannot be unable to walk, although perhaps it is unable to progress. I suggest that the phrase indicates, repetitively, a stalled labour resulting in the death of the foetus.
65 L. M. C. Weston, 'Women's Medicine, Women's Magic', *Modern Philology*, 92.3 (1995), 279–93 (p. 289).
66 Ibid., p. 283.

3

Overlap and overwriting in medical language for childbirth

Graveyards tell us that the thing most likely to kill a woman is childbirth or the complications surrounding it. Despite the fact that childbirth was the most pervasive cause of death for young women in early medieval England, there are remarkably few Old English remedies relating to childbirth. Few medical remedies offer any substantive help for a labouring woman in early medieval England. In some cases, these remedies seem to be written by and for people who don't really understand pregnancy or birth. The absence of such remedies does not occur under a single banner of malevolent silence, but rather through a series of sleights, some informed by ignorance, some by oversight, some by sheer carelessness and some by taboo. Compilers contemporary to the remedies as well as modern scholars help to erase and elide these remedies in a variety of ways, often by generalising remedies for women into a broad, capacious category. Through a careful attention to language, and by reading remedies across the corpus in conversation with one another, I disambiguate those remedies that are specific to childbirth, and those that are for other reproductive needs.

Part of the difficulty in examining the language for childbirth begins not with the manuscripts themselves, but rather with the nineteenth-century tools so intimately tied to the discipline of early English studies. These tools erase the reproductive bodies of women from the medical tradition in both literal and figurative ways. Early translators have a habit of glossing over the details of women's bodies; they are notoriously egregious in their desire to avoid the topic of and language around menstruation, a topic that medieval texts tie closely to women's health. Translators evade discussions of menstruation, even refusing to offer modern English translations of Old English, signalling a more general avoidance of language and ideas around women's reproductive health, which I have discussed briefly in prior chapters. For instance, the infamous first translator of the medical remedies, Thomas Oswald Cockayne, repeatedly uses Latin rather than offering a translation into English in discussions of menstruation. As an example, in an awkward mid-phrase translation into Latin, Cockayne renders the Old English from *LBIII* – 'Wiþ þon þe wifum sie forstanden hire monaþgecynd' – as 'In case mulieribus menstrua suppressa sunt', rather than 'In case a woman's menstruation is obstructed'.[1] The decision to begin the phrase in modern English and then shift to Latin allows him to avoid vernacular language for menstrual concerns.[2] The Latin is a way of creating distance from the distasteful processes of women's reproductive bodies, and effacing a process that is natural but is treated as outside the interest or comfort of his academic audience.[3] This practice of obscuring the feminine is embedded in the earliest dictionaries and translations that form the foundation of the discipline of Old English studies.

Similarly, the wide range of dictionary definitions available in the *DOE* demonstrates that no single Old English word universally signals only childbirth, or only conception, or only pregnancy, or only fertility.[4] According to the dictionary, these Old English words overlap, and that overlap contributes to both our present-day lack of understanding of women's bodies and the remedies. Even *beorþor*, a word that most closely resembles our contemporary language for birth, despite the rarity of its usage, does not provide a concrete semantic divide between pregnancy and childbirth, as it signifies a 'pregnancy, gestation', 'childbirth, delivery', and 'fetus, offspring'.[5]

The terms that most frequently appear in reference to birth-like activities are *cennan, geeacnian, geberan* and *afedan*. Each of these terms is used widely in the broader corpus of Old English, with hundreds of occurrences for each term. As most widely used terms do, these terms require many subdefinitions in order to account accurately for differences in usage across the corpus. The chart in Table 3.1 includes the most relevant definitions regarding reproduction, and demonstrates that each of these terms might mean almost

Table 3.1 Definitions and occurrences of *geberan*, *cennan*, *afedan*, *geeacnian*

Old English word	Definition	DOE definition	Occurrences
geberan	'to carry'	1	105[a]
	'to bring'	2	
	'fetus'	7	
	'to carry a child in the womb'	8	
	'to bring forth, bear'	9	
	'to conceive'	9.e	
cennan	'to create'	A.3	1976[b]
	'to generate'	A	
	'to bear, bring forth'	A.1	
	'to be pregnant'	A.1.b	
	'to conceive'	A.2	
	'genitals'	A.2.d	
	'to procreate'	A.4	
	'to multiply, propagate'	A.4.b	
	'to make known, declare'	B	
afedan	'to maintain, nourish life'	1	214[c]
	suckling/nursing a child	1.a.i	
	nurturing or raising a child	2	
	'to bring forth or produce a child'	3	
	'to be born'	3.a	
	'to nourish a child in the womb; to gestate to full term'	3.b	

Table 3.1 (Cont.)

Old English word	Definition	DOE definition	Occurrences
geeacnian	'to increase, to conceive'	4	180[d]
	'to be big with child'	5	
	'to be in labour'	6	

Notes:
[a] 'Geber ...' in a search of the *DOE English Web Corpus*, 15 July 2023. Beran, which has some definitional overlap, occurs about 950 times. The moments of overlap are discussed later in this chapter.
[b] 'Cen ...' in a search of the *DOE Web Corpus*, 15 July 2023. This search accounts for variations in spelling that include *acennan* and its forms.
[c] 'Afed ...' in a search of the *DOE Web Corpus*, 15 July 2023. *Fedan*, which includes some overlap and is also used in the medical texts, although not remedies relevant to this chapter, occurs about 375 times.
[d] 'Geac ...' in a search of the *DOE Web Corpus*, 15 July 2023.

anything along the range of reproductive experiences. Each term has been used to describe the entirety of the reproductive process, from intercourse, to conception, to pregnancy, to childbirth, and in some cases even to the nursing of a born child. The job of a dictionary is to offer all possible definitions; the job of the translator is to decide which definitions are most suitable. But most translations do not attend to the category of women's remedies at large, and so efficiently decide on their use without considering the specific diction of this precise group of remedies. In the past, scholars have been content to conjecture by content – content that is not always illuminating – but what I offer in the following sections is a thorough analysis of the occurrence of terms for childbearing wherein the logic of individual occurrences is balanced against the systemic use of the terms.

The language that we use for medical experiences and procedures matters, just as the language that we use for who experiences these medical needs has serious consequences. Although this book follows its medieval sources in identifying women as the people who need care for their reproductive needs, people in the present moment who do not identify as women continue to require medical treatment for concerns having to do with the possession of a uterus. When we identify this kind of medicine as 'women's medicine' only, we exclude many people, and far too many people therefore do not receive the medical care they need and deserve. Just as the medical language for childbirth and other reproductive concerns in the early Middle Ages matters, so too does the language we use now for who should and can have access to medicine.

By examining the language of reproduction and fertility in its specific medical context, I argue for a linguistic pattern that distinguishes specific reproductive problems with distinct uses of language in medical texts. In the medical texts, *afedan* remedies facilitate conception and maintaining a pregnancy after miscarriage, while *geeacnian* remedies are specific to conception. Both *cennan* and *geberan* signify childbirth explicitly. In determining these discrete categories, I work to undo the damage of clustering all of women's reproductive remedies into an expansive category that can be easily dismissed or overread.

Afedan: Therapeutic post-miscarriage pregnancy remedies

While *afedan* is, in some ways, the least overladen of the verbs associated with childbirth, it has been simplified to the detriment of a full understanding of these remedies. *Afedan* means, on a literal level, 'to feed', but might be more effectively read here as 'to nourish'.[6] Of course, even the idea of nourishment is difficult to compartmentalise in reproductive terms. Each phase requires nourishment, from the body hoping for fertility (and, likely in early England, lacking sufficient nourishment), to the body that has conceived but must nourish the foetus as it grows, to the postpartum body, which must nourish the newborn baby.

Lisa Weston argues that the three *afedan* remedies were purposely collected together as disparate remedies united by their use of the term *afedan*:

> The woman's inability to *afedan hire cild* may be variously translated 'nourish her child in her womb', 'bring her child to term', and 'nurse her child' after its birth. Though E. V. K. Dobbie, Felix Grendon, Godfrid Storms and J. H. G. Grattan, and Charles Singer all edit them as one, the evidence would suggest that the scribe has in fact gathered together three separate but related remedies. Their shared

rubric subsumes all of childbearing from conception to weaning, the entire period during which the child depends upon the nurturance and potency of its mother's body. While the manuscript commonly collects alternative remedies under repeated headings, it does not elsewhere conflate multiple complaints in this fashion. The conflation as well as the rubric implies that these are women's concerns, things beyond the male physician's domain.[7]

Weston diagnoses the same problem that I address in this chapter: that neither the learned medieval tradition nor the contemporary scholarly one attends fully to the language. However, she believes *afedan* stretches across the entirety of a pregnancy; instead, I suggest that it is specific to women who have lost pregnancies and seek healing for both their minds and bodies.

Afedan does not seem to mean the act of birth itself, although nourishment must both precede and follow it. In the previous chapter, I discussed remedies that promote fertility and conception, including one of the remedies that employs *afedan*. The *Lacnunga*'s *afedan* remedies, often about conception, are also remedies aimed at women who have experienced foetal loss. These are post-miscarriage fertility remedies, and so while they are not explicitly about birth, they are very much invested in the experience and trauma of childbirth.

A striking quality of the *afedan* remedies is their empathy for the women who might employ them; they are almost therapeutic as they encourage processes of grief and then hope. Perhaps this empathetic approach drove the early scholarly impulse to dismiss them as superstitious – ironic, because they might well have been the most psychologically efficacious remedies for suffering women. I previously discussed at length the *afedan* remedy that calls for the woman to step over a grave, then her partner, and finally declare her pregnancy at church. The remedy begins by identifying its intended recipient as 'Se wifman se hire cild afedan ne mæg' ('The woman who cannot carry to term her child').[8] The remedy itself makes clear its goal, for the three phases of the remedy move from the barren body to the newly pregnant body, to the body secure in its pregnancy: it is not until the woman has reached this final stage that the remedy is complete. The trouble she faces is made manifest in the ritual phrase she is to use as she steps over her husband: 'Up ic gonge, ofer þe stæppe, mid cwican cild, nalæs mid cwelendum, mid fulborenum, nalæs mid fægan' ('Up I go, over you I step with a living child, not with a dying one, with a fully gestated child, not with a doomed one').[9] The difference between a woman who cannot and a woman who can *afedan* her foetus is that the child of the former is *cwelendum* (dead) and *fægan* (doomed/fated); the woman for whom this remedy works has a foetus that is *cwican* (quickened) and *mid fulborenum* (fully gestated). This phrase might suggest that only a born child shows the nature of *afedan*, but the remedy ends when 'seo modor gefele þæt þæt bearn si cwic' ('the mother feels that the child is quickened'). A child is *afedan*, then, at quickening. After quickening, the loss of a foetus is a different kind of problem. Therefore, the critical stage of the body that must be able to *afedan* occurs not in the moment of conception, necessarily, but rather it is a more prolonged process, one bound up with problems of infertility, but also with early pregnancy loss.

The second *afedan* remedy makes less clear the end goal, but instead focuses on the resolution of grief at the loss of a pregnancy. This remedy uses a parallel structure to the previous remedy in its opening phrase: it is for 'Se wifmon se hyre bearn afedan ne mæge' ('The woman who cannot carry to term her child').[10] The focus of the remedy is, indeed, the woman who cannot nourish her foetus, but the remedy seems to concentrate not on how she can acquire or nourish a new foetus, but rather on how she can stop mourning a dead one. The first step of this remedy calls for her to gather earth from her dead child's grave: 'genime heo sylf hyre agenes cildes gebyrgenne dæl' ('she should take a portion of her own child's grave').[11] Because the remains of young children are so delicate, few remain in graveyards, and archaeologists cannot be certain regarding burial practices for young children or miscarried foetuses; the remedy makes unclear the state of the child being mourned, so the context of this remedy with the previous one suggests a child dead from pregnancy loss. It is also possible that *afedan* could be about a postbirth problem of nourishment, or a failure to nurse or thrive. But again, the remedy does not seek to help the woman conceive again, but rather encourages her to part with her grief. The mechanism for this process is the ritual selling of grief, for she is to take the portion of the grave and 'wry æfter þonne on blace wulle ond bebicge to cepemannum ond cweþe þonne: "Ic hit bebicge, ge hit bebicgan þas sweartan wulle, ond þysse sorge corn"' ('afterwards, wrap it in black wool and sell it to traders and then say: "I sell it; you sell it; this dark wool and the kernels of this sorrow"'). She is literally to wrap up the dirt in mourning cloth, and to sell that cloth to a trader.[12] The idea here is not to give away grief, but instead to sell it someone – to receive something in return for the grief. The notion of the trader invokes the idea of someone who travels and will carry away purchased grief.

It is unclear what the woman receives for the grief she sells, but the grief itself, the pieces of the grave, become *corn*, a word that can mean kernel, but also corn, or even grain. The grave dirt becomes something productive and fruitful, despite its affiliation with *sorge* (sorrow), once it has been sold. As Christina Lee notes, in thinking about the black wool necessary for the remedy,

> The whole process is clearly a ritual for a parent in severe distress, and may have been a symbolic act of separation. Miscarriage is quite common in the first twenty weeks of pregnancy, but whereas it is emotionally distressing today, for Anglo-Saxon parents, childlessness had far bigger consequences.[13]

Lee means here that families' economic well-being depended on their ability to produce and raise productive children, not that either modern-day or medieval grief contains less value. Miscarriage today remains a taboo subject, but its medieval consequences might be financially as well as emotionally devastating for a woman and her family. This remedy raises the spectre of economic exchange, but it does so in the service of trading away a grief that seems to be preventing a person from moving forward. This remedy for *afedan* focuses not on new life, but literally on the *wifmon*, the woman being addressed here, and her mental well-being.

The final *afedan* remedy has been widely read as a nursing remedy; I argue that it is, rather, primarily a post-miscarriage pregnancy remedy. It uses an opening phrase similar to the previous two remedies: 'Se man se ne mæge bearn afedan' ('The woman who cannot carry to term her child').[14] This opening provides little information regarding the true nature of the remedy, so *afedan* here might well suggest the literal feeding of an already-born child, or it might mean the nurturing of a foetus by a woman who has struggled to secure her pregnancy previously. Translators have used the content of the remedy to direct their translations, thus Niles and D'Aronco render the translation here as 'nurture', parallel to their translations in the previous remedies.[15] Lisa Weston argues that this remedy 'aids the woman who cannot breastfeed her child'.[16] This choice is likely dictated by the content of the remedy, and specifically by its use of milk as an ingredient:

> Se wifman ... nime þonne anes bleos cu meoluc on hyre handæ ond gesupe þonne mid hyre muþe, ond gange þonne to yrnendum wætere ond spiwe þærin þa meolc, ond hlade þonne mid þære ylcan hand þæs wæteres muð fulne ond forswelge; cweþe þonne þas word:
>
> 'Gehwer ferde ic me þone mæran maga þihtan. Mid þysse mæran mete þihtan. Þonne ic me wille habban ond ham gan.'
>
> Þonne heo to þan broce ga, þonne ne beseo heo no, ne eft þonne heo þanan ga; ond þonne ga heo in oþer hus oþer heo ut ofeode, ond þær gebyrge metes.
>
> [The woman ... should take milk of a cow of one colour in her hand and then sip it with her mouth, and then go to running water and spit the milk into it, and then ladle up a mouthful of the water with the same hand and swallow it; then speak these words:
>
> 'Everywhere I myself have carried the splendid strong son by means of this splendid, strong meat. I will have him and go home.'
>
> When she goes to the brook, then she should not look back, nor again when she goes from there, and then she should go into a house other than that from which she went out, and there let her eat meat.][17]

The consumption and spitting of milk contribute to the interpretation of a more literal kind of feeding of a child. The ritual spitting out of the household milk, although of a cow and not of a woman, works as a kind of disavowal of the insufficient milk, and the consumption of the surging ('yrnendum') water suggests a replacement of low milk production with an endlessly flowing supply.[18] The recited phrase furthers this reading, as it suggests a timescale where the woman has carried ('ferde') her strong son everywhere, and now wishes to have/keep ('habban') him, which might suggest a successful end to a pregnancy, but a struggle in the early days of life.

However, this remedy functions in precisely the same way the previous *afedan* remedies do: as a remedy to promote pregnancy until quickening. Indeed, I suspect that it is only the use of milk as an ingredient that suggests to readers it is about nursing as opposed to pregnancy.[19] Much of the content echoes the same kind of extruding of the past that the previous two remedies employ. Just as they call for the leaping over the grave and the selling of grave dirt, here the idea of failed nourishment is ritually discarded in the spitting of milk into the river. The taking up of new water in the same hand – 'ond hlade þonne mid þære ylcan hand þæs wæteres, muð fulne ond forswelge' ('and then ladle up a mouthful of the water with the same hand and swallow it') – turns the mouth, emptied of milk, into a receptacle for something new and fresh and living. We might read the mouth, asymptotically, as a uterus, emptied of a lost child and now perhaps newly pregnant with a foetus not yet quickened. If we read in this way, then the ritual language for carrying and keeping a child refers not to keeping the child alive after birth, but rather to keeping the pregnancy, and strengthening the foetus into a 'mæran maga þihtan. Mid þysse mæran mete þihtan' ('splendid strong son by means of this splendid, strong meat'). Grattan translates *magaþihtan* as 'stomach-sturdy one', which might refer to the nourishment of the child, but seems equally like to suggest that the child remain sturdy inside his mother's womb.[20] Thus, *afedan* works in the same way as the previous remedies, suggesting the nurturing of a precarious pregnancy in those months after conception but prior to quickening.

The final steps of the remedy, where the woman turns from the water without looking back and returns to a different house in order to nourish herself, perform the manoeuvre of symbolically treating the mouth as uterus. Here, the first home must be ritually abjected and thus figured as the inhospitable uterus: 'Þonne heo to þan broce ga, þonne ne beseo heo no, ne eft þonne heo þanan ga; ond þonne ga heo in oþer hus oþer heo ut ofeode, ond þær gebyrge metes' ('When she goes to the brook, then she should not look back, nor again when she goes from there, and then she should go into a house other than that from which she went out, and there let her eat meat'). In not returning to the first home to literally feed herself, the woman symbolically disavows the failed domestic space, and replaces it with something new. She cannot leave behind her actual uterus, but by using both mouth and home as proxy, as symbolic of the function of the uterus, places of home and nourishment, she can ritually refigure her body as a refuge capable of sustaining a foetus.

What these remedies share is a focus on the grieving and fearful mother, a woman who has lost, or fears to lose, her pregnancy. As Jones and Olsan beautifully note,

> Moreover, the focus in these Anglo-Saxon rituals is not on the last states of labor and delivery, rather on successful generation and gestation ... These performative acts impact her motherhood directly, creating the framework for success, where failure is a recognized likelihood or even a past reality. The verbal formulas name the worst fears, while performance of the stepping, selling, and sipping rituals persuades through words and bodily acts that something not only can be done, but has been done that creates a new reality. The last ritual of taking the milk, going to the stream silently, and taking food at a friend's house suggests that other people, most likely women, were aware and supportive of that ritual, as the presence of a sleeping husband is essential in the second set of stepping verses.[21]

The *afedan* remedies, collected together purposely, united by their use of common language, and a common referent, work to give hope and solace to women. They remind women that they are part of communities, and seek to reintegrate women into these communities as they publicly announce their happy news in church, sell away their grief and sit at table in their friends' homes, hopeful for safe pregnancies and the ability to nourish and sustain a quickened foetus. Thus the *afedan* remedies serve as remedies for psychological healing after miscarriage or other infant loss, rather than physical remedies for the womb.

Geeacnian: Remedies for conception

Whereas *afedan* refers to a specific portion of pregnancy, *geeacnian* is used almost exclusively to describe the problems and processes of conception. Despite the *DOE*'s assertion that this term can suggest being in labour, the only occurrences of this word in the medical texts that suggest a possibility other than conception are mirrored in parallel texts that use alternative language. Many of the *geeacnian* remedies were fully discussed in the previous chapter, so I will not repetitively explicate them here. Instead, I examine the patterns of language used for this particular aspect of reproduction, and demonstrate that in the *OEM*, it exclusively means conception.

In the *OEM*, *geeacnian* introduces remedies that are clearly linked to conception. There can be no question that the remedy using hare's stomach is for conception, as it requires consumption of the concoction prior to coitus:

> Wif to geeacnigenne: haran cyslybb feower penega gewæge syle on wine drincan þam wife of wife, and þam were of were, and þonne don hyra gemanan, and æfter þon hy forhæbben; þonne hraþe geeacnað heo, and for mete heo sceal sume hwyle swamma brucan and for bæð smyrenysse; wundorlice heo geeacnaþ.

> [To conceive a female: give four pennies' weight of the dried stomach of a hare to drink in wine, the female's for the woman, the male's for the man. Then they should have sexual intercourse, and after this they should abstain. Then she will conceive right away. And for a while she should take mushrooms for food, and in the place of a bath, ointments. She will conceive wonderfully.][22]

The remedy uses variations of *geeacnian* thrice, emphasising its goal, and including a postcoital treatment that suggests an understanding of conception as a process that exceeds the initial deposit of sperm. In its first use of *geeacnian*, in the introductory phrase, we are told that this is a remedy 'wif to geeacnigenne' ('to conceive a female'). This remedy is aimed at a time at the beginning of the process of reproduction – a time prior to pregnancy. The remedy explicitly commands the couple to engage in intercourse, after which it declares 'þonne hraþe geeacnað heo' ('*then* she will conceive right away' (emphasis mine)). The remedy offers a timeline: if a couple want to conceive, here is how they should proceed. If they time things correctly, then conception will occur; it is clear that here the remedy is not for the facilitation of birth, but rather for the beginning point of a pregnancy. In its final use of *geeacnian*, the remedy reiterates the quality of the conception that will occur, suggesting 'wundorlice heo geeacnaþ' ('she will conceive wondrously') if she applies the correct treatment to facilitate her conception of a daughter. As I discuss more fully in Chapter 4, conception is understood to be a continuing process, with ensoulment of girls occurring at ninety days post-intercourse (forty days for boys). Therefore the treatment of the body during what we now would understand as early pregnancy was part of the long process of conception in the early Middle Ages.

Not all remedies are as explicit about their outcomes as this one, and so thinking about this term as governing the group of remedies can help make sense of remedies that do not offer immediate clarity. For example, the *OEM* remedy for a speciality deer bone indicates its goal only through the verb *geeacnian*: 'Wið wifes geeacnunge: ban bið fonden on heortes heortan, hwilum on hrife, þæt ylce hyt gegearwað; gif ðu þæt ban on wifmannes earm ahehst, gewriðest scearplice, hræþe heo geeacnað' ('For a woman's conception: a bone may be found in the deer's heart, or sometimes in its womb, they have the same result; if you hang this bone on the woman's arm, bind it firmly, she will conceive right away').[23] The introductory phrase parallels that in the remedy for hare's stomach: 'wið wifes geeacnunge' ('for a woman's conception'). Nothing in the ingredients – the deer bone – offers an obvious statement about the expected result of the remedy, although perhaps the potential location of the bone in the womb might suggest general reproductive function. The conclusion of the remedy, where *geeacnian* is repeated, uses only vocabulary to account for the desired outcome. The remedy suggests that the wearing of this bone on the arm will help the woman in that 'hræþe heo geeacnað' ('she will conceive right away'). 'Hræþe' here can give us at least a hint about the meaning of *geeacnian*: it is likely not about general pregnancy, but rather focuses on the initiating moment of conception.

Two small elements of the remedy indicate that it is about conception rather than childbirth: first, the location of the bone, and second, the notion of the binding up of the body. The potential location of the bone in the deer's womb mimics the concept of something foreign, removable, placed in the womb of the woman. The wearing of this bone then works as a talisman for conception, for the filling of the womb. Second, the binding on of this bone parallels the symbolic notion of binding and loosening that is a part of the dialogue around menstruation, pregnancy and childbirth. Excess menstrual flows are to be 'bound up', and conception is the ultimate binding up of menstrual flow. Childbirth, oppositely, calls on the loosening and release of bonds.[24] Therefore, the tying on of the remedy, an item specifically found inside a womb, mimics the binding up of the seed in the womb, and indicates the remedy's focus on conception rather than birth.

The final remedy that makes use of *geeacnian*, however, demonstrates the semantic slide of the language around childbirth and conception. The main introductory clause for the *OEH* coriander remedy uses *cennan* – 'Wið þæt wif hrædlice cennan mæge' ('So that a woman may give birth quickly') – however, it inscrutably shifts to a form of *geeacnian* mid-remedy, as if the author is uncertain about what language more aptly describes what is to be treated.[25] One of the stranger (and less practical) remedies, it calls for an unlikely kind of assistance:

> genim þysse ylcan coliandran sæd, endlufon corn oððe þreottyne, cnyte mid anum ðræde on anum clænan linenan claþe, nime ðonne an man þe sy mægðhades man, cnapa oþþe mægden, ond healed æt þam wynstran þeo neah þam gewealde, ond sona swa eall seo geeacnung gedon beo, do sona þone læcedom aweg, þy læs þæs innoðes dæl þæræfter filige.

> [take this same coriander seed, eleven or thirteen seeds, knot them with a thread to a clean linen cloth, then take a person who is a virgin, boy or girl, and hold at the left thigh near the genitals, and immediately as soon as all the birthing is done, take the remedy away immediately, unless a portion of the intestines follow thereafter.][26]

The remedy calls for the attaching to the body of a small bag of coriander seeds, but unlike the other *geeacnian* remedies, it does not call for the remedy to be bound to the body, but rather for it to be held against the (extreme) upper thigh of the person seeking to give birth, *cennan*. However, in the latter part of the remedy, the author functionally shifts the verb *geeacnian* into its noun form, suggesting that the virgin must immediately remove the herbs 'sona swa eall seo geeacnung gedon beo', which I translate as 'immediately as soon as all the birthing is done', repeating the word immediately to mimic the repetition of 'sona' in order to indicate urgency.[27] Despite the use of *geeacnian*, which elsewhere in the remedies means 'conception', here that meaning seems almost impossible in practical terms, and to keep that translation here would be pedantic and disingenuous. One cannot imagine a virgin – either a boy or a girl – holding a cloth bag of herbs on a woman's upper thigh near the genitals during an act of conception, nor does it seem likely that a woman would extrude her organs after conception without removal of the bag.

The use of *geeacnian* alongside *cennan* in this remedy might have various explanations. Perhaps *geeacnian* is yet another general term with no distinct meaning, or perhaps the scribe of this manuscript was not well acquainted with distinctions in medical language around birth. The pool of evidence here is small, and so both are reasonable conclusions. If *geeacnian* indeed is the medical term for conception, as the previous evidence suggests, its occurrence here reveals a lack of knowledge on the part of the author, who might well fail to understand (or to care about) the difference between remedies for conceiving and giving birth, in fact seeing these two distinct medical processes as part and parcel of a larger unnameable, generalisable whole.

What makes me more certain that *geeacnian* is not a general term is the parallel remedy in *LBIII*, a remedy that does not use *geeacnian* in any part of the remedy. It begins by suggesting that it is 'To þon ilcan' ('For the same') disorder as the remedy that precedes it, a disorder that is expressed almost identically to the *OEH* remedy above: 'Wiþ þon þe wif ne mæge bearn acennan' ('In case a woman cannot give birth to a child').[28] Like the *OEH* remedy, it uses *cennan* to introduce the problem, but unlike the *OEH* remedy, it uses this verb throughout the remedy:

> Bind on þæt winstre þeoh up wiþ þæt cennende lim nioþowearde beolonan oþþe .XII. corn cellendran sædes and þæt sceal don cniht oþþe mæden. swa þæt bearn sie acenned do þa wyrta aweg þy læs þæt innelfe utsige.
>
> [Bind to the left thigh up against the genitals, the lower part of henbane, up to twelve grains of coriander seed, and that will make a boy or girl, whichever the child might be, be born; take the remedy away so that the internal organs do not come out.][29]

Where *OEH* uses the noun form *geeacnung* to indicate the end of the birthing process, here the scribe retains the verb 'acenned' and shifts the participation of the boy or girl from active contributor in the remedy to recipient of it: the child does not help with the birth, but rather is the child who is being born. Perhaps the *LBIII* is a superior version of an existing remedy, whereas the *OEH* version is garbled, or perhaps the *OEH* version is written by someone who does not understand at all what it is he is writing, and does not seem to understand that there is an appreciable difference between *cennan* and *geeacnian*. The latter seems more likely because of the shift of the child in the remedy from assistant to recipient, and the manner of application of the remedy from holding and removing to binding and then loosening. The *LBIII* remedy retains a consistency of language, clearly articulating that this odd remedy is for birth, not for conception.

Geeacnian is a term most frequently associated with the language and ideologies of conception. But this remedy operates contrary to remedies for conception, invoking the binding of a foetus to the womb, as opposed to the loosening of the connection so that the baby might be born. The odd occurrence of a term for conception in a remedy for childbirth may reveal confusion or unfamiliarity with women's reproductive processes on the part of a scribe. The compressed range of Old English language for reproduction, and the inconsistency in its use in this particular case, reflect a general discomfort or disregard for reproductive problems that is visible in the paucity of remedies for women at all, and for childbirth in particular. And yet, despite the strangeness of this remedy and its two versions, both use forms of the verb *cennan* to mean birth and not conception.

Cennan: Remedies for childbirth

Cennan is likely the least contentious of the reproductive terms, and seems to mean 'giving birth' almost exclusively and across multiple genres. Even in texts that are explicitly for conception, the term *cennan* indicates that aspect of birth necessary to support the outcomes of the conceptive remedy. The prognostics, as discussed in Chapter 2, consistently use this term, but do so in such a way as to refocus on that which is being born as opposed to she who is giving birth. The remedies direct attention oppositely, appropriate to their function to facilitate birth, and retain their focus on the birthing woman.

In the prognostics, there is no doubt that *cennan* means to give birth, or even to be born. For each day of the month, and the corresponding personality trait, the author uses the word *acennan*. Each of the dates in the birth lunarium begins with a numerically appropriate variation of the stock phrase 'Gif he biþ on tweigra nihta acenned' ('[if he is born on the second night']).³⁰ Consistently throughout all of the lunaria, *acenned* functions as the term for birth or being born on a particular date. In each case, the passive construction of the verb phrase moves our attention away from the person giving birth to the person being born. The child who is born is forever marked by this process. He is a passive recipient of birth; meanwhile, the active participant, the mother, remains entirely absent. This direction away from the mother's action and to the child is paralleled in literary texts that feature mothers. Mary Dockray-Miller suggests that in *Genesis A* the text provides 'lexical evidence for the subsuming of feminine, maternal work into masculine terminology', largely because of its connections with legal discourse: '*cennan* can imply the jural act of producing an heir, not the physical, maternal act of labor and delivery of a newborn infant'.³¹ Thus, while *cennan* works as a standard term for childbirth, its associations across the literary paradigm shift attention away from the body of the birthing woman, and to the heir she produces or the man for whom she produces this heir. The sheer volume and regularity of the usage of this term reify it as a standard term for childbirth, not conception or even reproduction more generally.

In the two *OEM* remedies for conception, the word *cennan* indicates birth, even as other language in the remedies conveys their primary purpose as the conception of male children. The outcome of the remedy cannot be known until after the birth of the child. That is, the remedy relies on the successful production – and not just conception – of a male child, and that is why *cennan* appears in them.³² These remedies, discussed more fully in the previous chapter, occur sequentially, and both use hare as an ingredient: 'To þan þæt wif cenne wæpned cild: haran hrif gedryged and gesceafen oððe gegniden on drinc drincen butu; gif þæt wif ana hyt drinceþ, ðonne cenð heo androginem; ne byþ þæt to nahte, naþer ne wer ne wif' ('So that a woman may give birth to a male child: let them both drink hare's womb, dried and scraped or crushed in a drink; if the woman alone drinks it, then she will give birth to an androgynous child, that is as nothing, neither man nor woman'). Niles and D'Aronco translate 'cenne' as 'conceive' and 'cenð' as 'generate'; these choices are reasonable given the content of the remedy, and yet do not account for the nuance of the term *cennan* in its wider medical context.³³ Given the logic of the remedy, and its choice of *cennan* instead of *geeacnian*, which it uses elsewhere,[34] then we can acknowledge that this remedy is about not merely what is conceived – although the instructions in the remedy must be performed as part of conception – but, more importantly, what is produced via childbirth.[35] Therefore, although the remedy itself is not about the facilitation of birth, the word *cennan* refers to birth and not conception in this context.

The medical remedies refocus *cennan* on the literal act of birth and birthing, emphasising the woman as the main actor of the verb. This is true for the *cennan* remedies discussed above, which clearly indicate that the woman who uses the remedy is attempting to give birth. In both of those remedies, the caveat that the leechdom must be removed 'þy læs þæt innelfe utsige' ('so that the internal organs do not come out')[36] solidifies their function as remedies where *cennan* means the expulsion of a foetus, not its conception.

The clarity of this coriander remedy in both *OEH* and *LBIII* can help us to understand the parallel remedies for wild carrot also extant in both texts. The remedies for wild carrot are relatively simple, with the one from *LBIII* calling for the woman to eat and drink the brewed wild carrots, while *OEH* calls for her to bathe herself with the solution (Table 3.2). *LBIII* suggests that the

Table 3.2 Remedy for wild carrot in *LBIII* and *OEH*

LBIII 37.1	*OEH* 82.1
Wiþ þon þe wif ne mæge bearn acennan. Nim feldmoran nioðowearde wyl on meolcum and on wætre do begea emfela sele etan þa moran and þæt wos supan.[a]	Feldmoru/pastinaca siluatica: Wið þæt wifmen earfuðlice [earfoþlice] cennen genim þas wyrte þe we pastinacam siluaticam nemdun, seoð on wætere, syle þonne þæt se man hyne þær mid beðige, he bið gehæled.[b]
[In case a woman cannot give birth to a child: take the lower part of wild carrot, boil in milk and in water, use the same amount of each, give the roots to eat and the liquid to sip.]	[Wild carrot or parsnip: for a woman who has difficulty in giving birth; take this herb we call *Pastinaca siluatica*, seethe it in water, give it so that the person can bathe [her]self with it, [she] will be healed.]

Notes:
[a] Cockayne, *Leechdoms*, Vol. II, p. 328 (37.1).
[b] Niles and D'Aronco, *Anglo-Saxon Medical Texts*, Vol. I, p. 196 (82.1).

remedy is for a woman who 'ne mæge bearn acennan' ('cannot give birth to a child'), whereas *OEH* suggests the remedy is meant to treat 'wifmen earfuðlice [earfoþlice] cennen' ('a woman with difficulty giving birth'). Aside from this introductory language, little in these remedies reveals exactly what is being treated. The *OEH* only suggests of the person who experiences difficulty in *cennan* that 'he bið gehæled' ('she will be healed'). It seems strange to suggest that a woman might be healed of childbirth, although certainly a postpartum body might require healing.

In order to identify the function of this remedy, unclear from the contents of the remedy itself, we must use both the language of the manuscripts and what we know about these herbs. Wild carrot, otherwise known as Queen Anne's Lace, 'is known to have a purgative effect on the body', and carrot seeds are 'known to act as abortifacients'.[37] Given this contextual information, we can infer that *cennan* is not about conception; indeed, conception is contraindicated. Thus, if the known properties of carrot are associated with expulsion, it seems likely that these remedies seek both to facilitate birth and perhaps in some cases for other kinds of expulsion of the foetus.

Although the word *cennan* seems to indicate to its early medieval audience the goals of the remedy without requiring further explanation, the *OEH* remedy using fleabane provides a statement of outcomes. It uses a variation of the word *cennan* to explain the result of the remedy for *cennan*. This remedy leads with the familiar description of the malady, but it also explains the results: 'Conize: Gif wif cennan ne mæge nime þysse ylcan wyrt wos mid wulle, do on þa gycyndelican; sona heo þa cenningce gefremeþ' ('Fleabane/Spikenard: If a woman has difficulty giving birth, take this same plant soaked in wool, and put it on the genitals; immediately she will enact birth').[38] Anne Van Arsdall cleverly translates 'gefremeþ' as 'induce', wherein the whole phrase is rendered 'it will quickly induce birth', indicating her interpretation of this remedy.[39]

Gefremman generally means 'to promote, perfect, perform, commit', but by translating it as 'induce', Van Arsdall employs familiar contemporary medical language.[40] The Old English phrase, however, is not so clear as her translation might lead us to believe. Van Arsdall suggests the actor is the herb rather than the woman. For her, the subject of the phrase becomes 'it' rather than 'heo' (she), and the woman becomes the passive recipient of the action, whereas I suggest we can instead read the woman as the subject: 'sona heo þa cennincge gefremeþ' ('immediately she will enact birth').[41] The verb phrase is not easy to convey: *gefremman* is a widely used verb that can mean anything from 'to do good' to 'to make progress' to 'to commit a sin/perpetrate a crime'.[42] Whereas the sense of 'induce' is unique to the recipe according to the *DOE*, other definitions, including 'to activate (a man's) carnal desire (in a medical recipe)'[43] or, more generally, 'to effect a cure',[44] may help to indicate its function in this context. While it is plausible to identify the herb as that which activates, doing so renders the woman the passive recipient of activation. I suggest that her own active participation is equally possible, but in either case, linking *gefremman* and *cennan* indicates that this remedy works to begin labour and facilitate childbirth.

The circular linguistic logic of this remedy is part of the difficulty in interpreting it. The remedy tells us that it is for a woman who cannot *cennan*, and the result is that she will be able to *cennan*. This circularity does not help us determine what *cennan* means and if it refers specifically to birth or not. *Cennincge*, from *cenning*, occurs approximately thirty times in the corpus of Old English, frequently in Aldhelm, but also in *Genesis*, Ælfric and glosses; it occurs only this single time in the medical texts. Whereas its first definition is 'birth' according to the *DOE* (particularly in reference to the Virgin Birth), its second meaning is 'mother'.[45] This is a striking reversal of the jural aspect of *cennan*, which Dockray-Miller asserts invokes ideas of paternity and inheritance.[46] *Cennincge*, alternatively, works as an active verb, birth, enacted not by the father, but rather by the mother. She is synonymous with the act of birthing. Thus, when we consider the phrase 'cennincge gefremmeþ', the language demands that we render the mother as the actor: she who gives birth. The job of this herb is to empower the mother to activate her own labour, and to give birth.

Reading the five remedies that use the word *cennan* in conversation with one another reveals a consistency in methods and results: these five remedies are intended to facilitate childbirth (Table 3.3). They not only repeat the same verb, but their phrasing is strikingly similar, despite their existence in two different texts.[47] While each of these remedies uses similar phrasing and

Table 3.3 Language in remedies that use *cennan*

'Wið þæt wif hrædlice cennan mæge' (*OEH*)[a]	[So that a woman may give birth quickly]
'Wiþ þon þe wif ne mæge bearn acennan' (*LBIII*)[b]	[in case a woman cannot give birth to a child]
'To þon ilcan' (*LBIII*)[c]	[for the same]
'Wið þæt wifmen earfuðlice [earfoþlice] cennen' (*OEH*)[d]	[If a woman has difficulty giving birth]
'Gif wif cennan ne mæge' (*OEH*)[e]	[If a woman cannot give birth]

Notes:
[a] Niles and D'Aronco, *Anglo-Saxon Medical Texts*, Vol. I, p. 243 (104.2).
[b] Cockayne, *Leechdoms*, Vol. II, p. 328 (37.1).
[c] Ibid., Vol. II, p. 328 (37.2, referencing 37.1).
[d] Niles and D'Aronco, *Anglo-Saxon Medical Texts*, Vol. I, p. 196 (82.1).
[e] Ibid., p. 292 (143.3).

repeats *cennan* as the desired main action, not all of the remedies are explicit about what a successful *cennan* looks like. The parallel nature of these phrases suggests that the remedies address a common problem; where individual remedies do not clarify the precise nature of the problem, reading them in the context of the remedies that *do* helps us to understand their purpose as a whole, and therefore to identify the correct medical interpretation of *cennan*.

(Ge)Beran: Unbinding pregnancy

Despite the fact that *beran* occurs over 900 times in the Old English Corpus at large, it occurs rarely in the medical corpus. As do most words that occur frequently in a range of genres, *beran* includes a wide range of meanings, including to carry, bear, transport and wear, as well as to bring forth. In fact, in the *DOE*, definitions for *beran* related to childbirth are the twelfth and thirteenth options listed, and they include 'to carry a child (acc.) in the womb';[48] as an adjective, meaning 'pregnant';[49] 'to bring forth, bear (someone / something acc.); in past participle: born';[50] and, in the laws, it is 'used to describe lawful or noble birth'.[51] The variation *geberan*, with only eighty occurrences, has a stronger connection with childbearing in the corpus at large, but both terms occur equally rarely in the medical corpus: once each.[52] Perhaps it is the vastness of usage of this term and its variants that makes it unsuitable for medical use: it simply means too much. It is overdetermined, and consequently difficult to use diagnostically.

The word *geberan* occurs in *Bald*'s 'Table of Contents', paired with other reproductive terms. Since we do not have the remedy itself, we are left to conjecture what the term might really mean in this context. *Bald* says: 'gif wif bearn ne mæge geberan, oþþe gif bearn weorþe dead on wifes innoþe, oððe gif hio cennan ne mæg' ('if a woman may not bear a child, or if a child becomes dead in a woman's womb, or if she may not give birth').[53] Banham and Voth translate *cennan* as 'to give birth', which implicitly suggests that *geberan* must mean something different.[54] 'To bear' makes sense, as the phrase is familiar to contemporary readers, but 'to bear' does not specify the particular dilemma faced by the woman who cannot do it. By a process of elimination, we can surmise that it does not mean 'stillbirth' or 'miscarriage', as the 'Table of Contents' gives specific language for that malady. If *cennan* means 'to give birth', then what might 'bearn ne mæge geberan' mean in practical medical terms? We have no remedy to help provide further information, and only one other occurrence in the medical corpus.

Despite differences in the manuscripts that contain *beran* and *geberan*, placing the terms side by side allows us to understand their medical function more clearly. The *Lacnunga* remedy that uses *beran* is notoriously difficult to interpret. Translators tend to brush over its garbled Latin invocation, leaving it in its original language rather than offering interpretation:[55] 'Gif wif ne mæge bearn beran/ Solue, iube, D(eu)s, ter, catenis'.[56] Voth translates it: 'If a woman cannot bear her child: Solue [Salve?], iube, Deus, ter, catenis'. Cockayne says inconclusively 'If a woman is not able to bear a child. *Hymnus*? Solvi iube/ Deus e catenis',[57] adding an instruction to sing that does not seem to be present in the manuscript. G. H. Brown argues that this formulation is a corruption of the phrase '"Solve iubente Deo terrarium Petre catenas" (Peter, release by God's command the chains of the world)',[58] and Cameron and Brown critique manuscript interventions taken by Grattan and Singer in order to make sense of difficult phrases like this one.[59] This phrase, therefore, has long caused editors and readers to move quickly past both the difficult language and the remedy itself, rather than to understand how this passage might have fitted into the corpus of remedies for women.

The Latin phrase is for release, for unbinding, and therefore for childbirth. 'Solve catenis' means 'release from chains'.[60] Despite the awkwardness of its grammar, the remedy calls for a plea to God for unchaining. Such an implication does not fit with the language around conception: what chains would require loosening in that situation? In Chapter 1, I showed that the remedies for ending excessive menstrual bleeding call for the binding up of the flow, and posited that calling for a flow to be released might suggest a wish *not* to be pregnant. If here the language calls for unbinding, then it cannot be a remedy for conception or pregnancy, both of which would be seeking to bind up a flow rather than to release one. Instead, the loosening of chains indicates the facilitation of childbirth, wherein literal body parts must loosen and soften in order to allow a child to be born. We might also think about the problem of painful contractions as the kind of chains binding a birthing body, and the desire for the loosening of those chains. This remedy is not for a general purpose: it is a childbirth remedy, not one for 'barrenness'.[61]

Despite the limited occurrences of *beran* in the medical corpus, the evidence from *Lacnunga* shows a strong affiliation with remedies for birth. *Beran* is a cipher in *Bald*, as we have only differentiation to determine its meaning, and lack any remedy that might demystify its use. Its occurrence in *Lacnunga* shows that while it might be reasonable to translate *Bald*'s phrase 'gif wif ne mæg bearn (ge)beran' as 'if a woman may not bear a child', the phrase more literally suggests 'if a woman cannot give birth to a child'. Despite the strong distinctions between the two medical texts in question, they posit the problem by using nearly identical language. Indeed, taken side by side, in addition to the language we begin to see that the only treatments for the problem of women who cannot *beran* are belief-based. Bald's header suggests that this malady can be treated by the wearing of a prayer, and *Lacnunga* by the speaking of one. Neither remedy requires any physical examination, or expertise in herbs or poultices. Indeed, they do not even require a solid knowledge of Latin, though likely they both require specific ritual phrases. And if the solution to the medical problem lies in ritual and repeated phrases, it seems probable that the phrasing of the problem itself, and the fact that it is parallel between two very different texts, is either a common-use phrase, or a textually formulaic one.

Conclusions

I suggested in the introduction to this chapter that six remedies were difficult to categorise in terms of their purpose. By virtue of the content alone, the goal of the remedy remains unclear, beyond the verb in its introductory clause. Even expanding to its manuscript context – that is, thinking about the remedy in the context of the remedies that surround it – does not always elucidate the goal of the remedy. Reframing the scope of this conversation by thinking about language across manuscripts, while also paying attention to the individual qualities of remedies and their contexts, clarifies the purposes and categories that define these remedies.

Disambiguating reproductive terms in their larger generic context means that we know with greater certainty the specific kinds of help remedies offered to parents, or to those who hoped to become parents. Doing so means that I can say that five remedies are for conception, with three of those five indicating the desired sex of the infant.[62] Two of those five employ the language of birth, because their desired result cannot be verified until after birth. Three remedies are for the maintenance of a pregnancy after miscarriage (one of these also invokes ideas of nursing a child postpartum).[63] Six remedies address actual childbirth.[64] The only remedy that remains difficult to categorise – the listing for *geberan* in *Bald*'s 'Table of Contents' – can be better understood by placing it in conversation with other texts that use the term. The *Lacnunga* Latin incantation for *beran* suggests that the *Bald* occurrence indicates childbirth, despite its placement in a clause that differentiates it from *cennan*, which may indicate a distinction between ritual remedies for childbirth and herbal responses.

Separating remedies into discrete categories matters, because birth is an entirely different process than conception. To suggest that treatments for each would be interchangeable is to diminish the value of a birthing person's body, and to make little of the processes by which so many young people died. Previous translations have forwarded the notion, whether purposely or not, that the medical texts did not distinguish between reproductive processes. Readers might well take the choices of dictionaries and translations as truth, rather than the consequence of social prohibitions about gendered bodies and their medical and reproductive needs. By attaching language *to* category, and questioning the tools of the discipline, we find a clearer sense of both language *and* category.

The results of this close attention to language show that the range of terms for reproductive problems in the medical texts matters. These terms hold discrete meanings. The semantic distinctions between them – regardless of whether they were used to treat everyday women, or even any women at all – demonstrate a more meaningful response to reproductive bodies than we have previously understood. Language is a powerful tool by which we can include or exclude bodies in terms of their medical treatment or an assessment of their value. In this book, I use the language of the texts to identify women as those who give birth; this gender binary is not a universal truth, and there are many people who give birth who do not identify as women. Using language as a tool to exclude such people has dangerous consequences for their lives and safety. At the heart of my work is the idea that language matters; just as we must carefully attend to the language that texts give us, and the categories such language constructs, so too must we question the ways in which contemporary language and reliance on traditional categories for the sake of their tradition erect barriers at the very real expense of people's lives.

Notes

1 Thomas Oswald Cockayne, *Leechdoms, wortcunning, and starcraft of early England. Being a collection of documents, for the most part never before printed, illustrating the history of science in this country before the Norman Conquest*, 3 vols (London: Longman, Green, Longman, Roberts and Green, 1864–66), Vol. II, pp. 330–1 (38.1). Other examples of this practice include the following: when the Old English of the *OEM* reads 'Wið wifes flewsan', he translates the phrase only as 'Ad mulieris fluxum' (Cockayne, *Leechdoms*, Vol. I, pp. 332 (1.6), 334 (2.4)), rather than the more literal translation of 'for a woman's flow', immediately thereafter giving a modern English translation for the remainder of the remedy. The same is true for the following remedy, where he translates 'Eft gif heo wylle þæt ðæt hyre

blodryne cyme to' (p. 332 (1.7)) as 'At si hoc optaverit, ut menstrua fluant' (p. 333), rather than 'again, if she wishes that her bloodflow should come on', followed thereafter by an English translation of the rest of the remedy. While it might be reasonable to assume that contemporary language for menstruation for his time was in fact Latin, there is no call to use Latin for the entirety of the introductory phrases of these remedies.

2 This kind of linguistic discomfort is part and parcel of the occlusion and abjection of women's bodies, a move that is not unique to Cockayne. In fact, Cockayne's intellectual nemesis, Joseph Bosworth, also turned to Latin to avoid the language around menstruation, translating 'monaþgecynd' as 'menstruum' in his dictionary, clarifying only by offering the Old English phrase (from the remedies) 'Gif wife to swiðe of flowe sio monaþgecynd' without further translation or discussion. Joseph Bosworth, 'mónaþ-gecynd', in *An Anglo-Saxon Dictionary Online*, ed. Thomas Northcote Toller, Christ Sean and Ondřej Tichy (Prague: Faculty of Arts, Charles University, 2014), https://bosworthtoller.com/23114 (accessed 3 January 2024). For more on the conflict between Cockayne and Bosworth, see Anne Van Arsdall, *Medieval Herbal Remedies: The Old English Herbarium and Anglo-Saxon Medicine* (London: Routledge, 2002), especially pp. 5–12.

3 In the 1960 introduction to Cockayne's *Leechdoms*, Charles Singer has no hesitation in designating certain parts of the medical tradition as distasteful, as when he lists the parts of Pseudo-Apuleius's text (what we call *OEM*), identifying one part as 'a disgusting little work on the badger' and the next 'an equally nauseating book on medicines derived from animals' (pp. xxi–xxii). It is clear that the judgemental hand of an academic mediator is not without bias, well past the nineteenth century.

4 Latin glosses do not provide any clear answers: while *beorþre* only glosses *feotu*, (foetus), and *afedde* glosses *confovere* ('to nurse, foster, cherish'), *geeacnian*, *geberan* and *cennan* gloss a much larger list of Latin terms each. *Geeacnian* glosses *concipit.i.*, *accipit*, *intellegit*, and *DOE* also notes the following correspondences: 'Lat. equiv. in ms: *accipere, addere, augere, augmentare, +concipere, intellegere, parturire; adicere*'. The *DOE* notes '*bajulare, concipere, gerere, gestare, ingerere, parere, parturire, +portare, sufferre; fetosus* (with *fecundus*), *fetus*' as terms equivalent to *geberan*, while it suggests '*creare, edere, eniti, generare, germinare, gignere, nasci, parere, parturire; genitalia = þa cennendan; nascentia*' for *cennan*. My point here is not exhaustively to examine each of these

Latin terms, but rather to demonstrate the truly remarkable range of Latin terms that these five Old English words work to transmit. Clearly Latin uses many different and precise terms for reproductive processes, but Old English condenses the range of these terms, and lacks differentiation.

5 *DOE*, 'beorþor', definitions 1.a, 1.b and 2. *Beorþor/byrþor* occurs only twenty-five times, three of which are in the remedies, although there may be more occurrences with some variation in spelling.

6 Mary Dockray-Miller uses the notion of postpartum *gefedan* to articulate the woman's contribution to the child: 'Only one of the three words that describes the births of Eve's children indicates Eve acting as maternal subject ... Fedan is the third verb in the poem that is translated "to beget", used to describe the birth of Seth, and it too occurs in the past participle (like cennan and (a)strienan) to obfuscate the physical maternal body that produces the child ... Adam is defined as the parent here ... but the verb literally means "feed" and other translations include "nourish" or "sustain". The connotations of this verb, unlike cennan and (a)strienan, point to the maternal body and the physical needs of the infant. Although the verb is a past participle, it reflects the Vulgate text in that it acknowledges the integral female contribution to childbearing.' Mary Dockray-Miller, 'Breasts and Babies: The Maternal Body of Eve in the Junius 11 *Genesis*', in Benjamin Withers and Jonathan Wilcox (eds), *Naked before God* (Morgantown: West Virginia University Press, 2003), pp. 221–56 (p. 243). She also notes: 'The Old English poet's unusual choice of fedan (why not repeat cennan or strienan, as the Vulgate repeats peperit?) forces the reader to acknowledge the physicality of children and their mothers ... Fedan equates nourishing with birthing, or with begetting, and although Eve is not mentioned in this sentence, the verb used subtly reminds the text's reader that the mother's body was an absolutely necessary part of birthing and feeding the child' (p. 243).

7 L. M. C. Weston, 'Women's Medicine, Women's Magic', *Modern Philology*, 92.3 (1995), 279–93 (pp. 282–3).

8 John P. Niles and Maria D'Aronco (eds and trans), *Anglo-Saxon Medical Texts*, Vol. I, *The Old English Herbal, Lacnunga, and Other Texts*, Dumbarton Oaks Medieval Library (Cambridge, MA: Harvard University Press, 2023), p. 510 (161). Niles and D'Aronco translate this 'The woman who cannot rear her child', which follows from Edward Thomas Pettit's notes about the remedy, where he comments upon this collection of remedies 'forming a group for problems in rearing a child'; 'A Critical Edition of the Anglo-Saxon *Lacnunga* of BL MS Harley 585', PhD thesis (King's College London, 1996), p. 47.

9 J. H. G. Grattan notes: 'By the first jingle the woman buries her misfortune in the earth … Then when she is again with child she reverses the former charm by stepping over a living man, instead of a dead one. Thus she acquires by sympathetic magic a virtue corresponding to the burden which she has lost.' J. H. G. Grattan, *Anglo-Saxon Magic and Medicine* (Oxford: Oxford University Press, 1952), p. 191.
10 Niles and D'Aronco, *Anglo-Saxon Medical Texts*, Vol. I, p. 512 (162).
11 Ibid.
12 Victoria Thompson suggests that the black cloth functions as 'an inverted reference to the white clothes of baptism'; *Death and Dying in Anglo-Saxon England* (Woodbridge: Boydell, 2004), p. 96. See also Christine Voth, 'Women and "Women's Medicine", Early Medieval England: From Text to Practice', in R. Trilling, R. Norris and R. Stephenson (eds), *Feminist Approaches to Anglo-Saxon Studies* (Amsterdam: Amsterdam University Press, 2023), pp. 279–316.
13 Christina Lee, 'Threads and Needles: The Use of Textiles for Medical Purposes', in Maren Clegg Hyer and Jill Frederick (eds), *Textiles, Text, Intertext: Essays in Honour of Gale R. Owen-Crocker* (Woodbridge: Boydell Press, 2016), pp. 103–17 (p. 114).
14 Niles and D'Aronco, *Anglo-Saxon Medical Texts*, Vol. I, p. 512 (163). Oddly, it identifies the sufferer using the generic *man*, rather than *wif* or *wifmon*, as the other two *afedan* remedies do, although it uses feminine pronouns thereafter.
15 Ibid., p. 513. Cockayne, in a strikingly attentive choice, translates it as 'Let the woman who cannot bring her child to maturity'; *Leechdoms*, Vol. III, p. 67 (103). For the second in the set of remedies, he translates it 'Let the woman who cannot bring up her bairn to maturity', and for the third, 'Let the woman who cannot rear her child' (p. 69 (103 and 104)).
16 Weston, 'Women's Medicine', p. 290. This essay explicitly expores the potential meaning of *afedan*, although she does not argue for a single meaning of the term, instead saying 'Individually, each of these charms empowers the childbearing woman and, indeed, the female community to which she belongs' (p. 291).
17 Niles and D'Aronco, *Anglo-Saxon Medical Texts*, Vol. I, pp. 513, 515.
18 As Voth says, 'Spitting the milk into running water symbolizes her own desire for her milk to flow'; 'Women and "Women's Medicine"', p. 296.
19 Peter Murray Jones and Lea T. Olsan note that 'Donald G. Scragg (Manchester: Manchester Centre for Anglo-Saxon Studies, 1989), 9–40 (esp. 24–25), thinks that afedan in this instance refers to nurture after, rather than before, birth, thus to lactation. The implication in the poetic lines that the fetus is fully formed and the rituals taking liquids and nourishment lend weight to this view.' 'Performative Rituals for

Conception and Childbirth in England, 900–1500', *Bulletin of the History of Medicine*, 89 (2015): 406–33 (p. 429 n. 65).
20 Grattan, *Anglo-Saxon Magic*, p. 191.
21 Jones and Olsan, 'Performative Rituals', pp. 429–30.
22 Niles and D'Aronco, p. 388 (5.14). This remedy follows two others that use *cennan* that invoke ideas of conception – unsurprising because the section is about hares. The shift in language is interesting.
23 Niles and D'Aronco, *Anglo-Saxon Medical Texts*, Vol. I, p. 380 (3.17).
24 For a discussion of the language around binding, see Tiffany Beechy, *The Poetics of Old English* (Farnham: Ashgate, 2011), particularly Chapter 3, 'Bind and Loose: Poetics and the Word in Old English Law, Charm, and Riddle', where she concludes 'The charms substitute the plane of language for the referential plane, allowing the order of poetic form to suffice, to stand in for an ordered cosmos' (p. 98). Megan Cavell also discusses the use of notions of binding in medicine, invoking the idea of the body being 'knotted together' (p. 195), but also two different notions of disease, where 'one refers conventionally to the binding of the body with pain and suffering, while the second turns convention on its head by referring to disease's attack on the body as the unlocking of a hoard'. *Weaving Words and Binding Bodies: The Poetics of Human Experience in Old English Literature* (Toronto: University of Toronto Press, 2016), p. 200.
25 Niles and D'Aronco, *Anglo-Saxon Medical Texts*, Vol. I, p. 234 (104.2).
26 Ibid., pp. 234, 236 (104.2).
27 *Geeacnung* can also mean foetus, or 'that which has been conceived', as I will discuss in greater depth in the next chapter. Here, however, that rendering does not seem accurate.
28 Cockayne, *Leechdoms*, Vol. II, p. 328 (37). Cockayne does not distinguish individual subsections here for this remedy, but a contemporary editor might do so, indicating them as 37.2 and 37.1.
29 Niles and D'Aronco, *Anglo-Saxon Medical Texts*, Vol. I, pp. 328, 330 (37.2).
30 Roy Liuzza, 'Birth Lunarium in English' (T15), in *Anglo-Saxon Prognostics: An Edition and Translation of Texts from London, British Library, MS Cotton Tiberius A.iii* (London: D. S. Brewer, 2011), p. 202.2. This pattern is also borne out in the 'General Lunarium' (T), which is in Latin, glossed with Old English. Here, *natus* is glossed repetitively as *acenned* in each of the thirty dates (pp. 125–46). Similarly, in the 'Birth Lunarium, Latin with English Gloss' (T5), the same glossing occurs (p. 158).

31 Dockray-Miller, 'Breasts and Babies', pp. 234–5.
32 These remedies have been discussed in greater depth in the previous chapter. I will primarily attend to their use of the word *cennan*, looking to the remedies to discuss their purposes in this respect.
33 Niles and D'Aronco, *Anglo-Saxon Medical Texts*, Vol. I, p. 387.
34 In *OEM*, both remedies 3.17 and 5.14 use variations of *geeacnian*; ibid., pp. 380, 388.
35 Niles and D'Aronco translate 'cenð' in the second remedy as 'to give birth to', rather than variations of 'to conceive': 'Eft, to þam ylcan: haran sceallan wife æfter hyre clænsunge; syle on wine drincan. þonne cenð heo wæpnedcild' ('Again, for the same: hare's testicles for the woman after her purification; give to drink in wine. She will give birth to a male child'); ibid., pp. 388–9 (5.13).
36 Cockayne, *Leechdoms*, Vol. II, pp. 328 (37.2).
37 John M. Riddle, *Contraception and Abortion from the Ancient World to the Renaissance* (Cambridge, MA: Harvard University Press, 1994), p. 58. Dioscorides, Pliny the Elder, Scribonius Largus and Constantine the African also identify carrot as an abortifacient and contraceptive, as noted in World Carrot Museum, 'Carrots and Their Contraceptive Purposes', www.carrotmuseum.co.uk/cont.html (accessed 9 August 2022).
38 Niles and D'Aronco, *Anglo-Saxon Medical Texts*, Vol. I, p. 292 (143.3).
39 Van Arsdall, *Medieval Herbal Remedies*, p. 212.
40 Bosworth, 'ge-fremman', in *An Anglo-Saxon Dictionary Online*, https://bosworthtoller.com/14424 (accessed 13 July 2023). The *DOE* also indicates this sense, perhaps following or perhaps inspiring Van Arsdall: 'cenninge gefremman "to bring about, i.e. induce, birth"'; Angus Cameron, Ashley Crandell Amos, Antonette diPaolo Healey et al., 'gefremman', in *Dictionary of Old English: A to I online* (Toronto: Dictionary of Old English Project, 2018), definition 3.a.viii. The only citation under this definition is this passage.
41 I respect Van Arsdall's translation and understand her changes as a way of handling a tricky verb phrase, despite my critique here. This critique is less about her translation than about the impact of language choices on the ways we perceive birth as either an active or passive affair. It is possible she takes 'heo' to refer to the herb rather than to the woman: there are instances wherein the same herbs are referred to as 'hyt' (p. 296 (145.1)) and 'heo' (p. 296 (145.2)), while others are both 'he' (p. 298 (146.1)) and 'hyt' (p. 298 (146.2)). I do not feel it is necessary to explain the 'heo' in this way, although I understand the choice.

42 *DOE*, definitions 1, 2, and 3.a.
43 *DOE*, 3.a.v.a. This sense is specific to the following remedy from *OEM*, p. 402 (9.8): 'weres wylla to gefremmanne: nime bares geallan ond smyre mid þone teors ond þa hærþan, þonne hafað he mycelne lust' ('to increase a man's desire to perform: take boar's gall and smear the penis and testicles with it; then he will have great lust').
44 *DOE*, 3.a.vii. This use is linked to occurrences in *Elene* and *The Wanderer*.
45 *DOE*, 'cennicge', definitions A.1 and A.2.
46 Dockray-Miller says 'The other possible meaning of cennan, however, tends to impart a "masculine" connotation to the word, despite the specifically maternal associations of giving birth. Cennan primarily means "to beget" or "to bear" ... but it can also mean to declare or to bring forth evidence in court'; Dockray-Miller, 'Breasts and Babies', p. 235.
47 *OEH* and *LBIII* have common remedies, which suggests a common source, but they do not share all of the same remedies; the remedy for fleabane is unique.
48 *DOE*, 'beran', 12.a.
49 *DOE*, 'beran', 12.b.
50 *DOE*, 'beran', 13.a.
51 *DOE*, 'beran', 13.c.
52 Like *beran*, *geberan*'s primary definition according to the *DOE* is 'to carry, bear', with a similar range of alternative definitions, but also means 'to bear fruit' (definition 7); works as a 'present participle glossing fetus "fruitful" or fetosus "prolific"' (7.b); can mean 'to carry (a child acc.) in the womb' (8) or 'to bring forth, bear young' (9.a); and is used to gloss 'concipere "to conceive"' (9.e).
53 Cockayne, *Leechdoms*, Vol. II, p. 172 (60).
54 I am grateful to Debby Banham and Christine Voth for sharing early drafts of their forthcoming Dumbarton Oaks edition of *Bald* with me; Debby Banham and Christine Voth (eds and trans), *Old English Medicine in British Library, Royal D. xvii*, Vol. II of *Anglo-Saxon Medical Texts*, Dumbarton Oaks Medieval Library (Cambridge, MA: Harvard University Press, forthcoming). Cockayne translates 'cennan' in this passage as 'may not bear a bairn, or if a bairn become dead in a womans inwards, or if she may not kindle or bring it into the light'; *Leechdoms*, Vol. II, p. 173.
55 Felix Grendon suggests it is one of several charms that made use of 'Christian formulas lacking a definite liturgical character'; 'The Anglo-Saxon Charms', *The Journal of American Folklore*, 22.84 (April–June 1909), 105–237 (p. 152).

56 Niles and D'Aronco, *Anglo-Saxon Medical Texts*, Vol. I, p. 508 (156). G. H. Brown describes the manuscript placement thus: 'The words appear in line 2 as "Solue iubedster catenis", with a capital S for Solue, indicating a major entry, and an erasure of two or three letters between the r and c'; G. H. Brown, 'Solving the "Solve" Riddle in BL, MS Harley 585', *Viator*, 18 (1989), 45–51 (p. 45). He further notes: 'What editors and commentators have not noted is that from fol. 179, line 10, to the end is an addition. Even a cursory examination of the addition demonstrates that it contains even more errors, solecisms, misspellings, misplacement of letters and words, erasures, odd abbreviations, and garbled Latin than the rest of the manuscript. The author has only a tenuous hold on the Latin language, and he or the scribe, if that is a different person, is careless' (p. 47).

57 Cockayne, *Leechdoms*, Vol. III, p. 64 (98).

58 Brown, 'Solving the "Solve" Riddle', p. 47. He suggests 'Peter's cult was widespread in England; more churches were dedicated to him there than to any other saint. An Anglo-Saxon charm calling upon this heavenly key-bearing authority of binding and loosing is entirely apposite, either for the binding of the womb to prevent miscarriage or the loosing of the womb to allow childbirth (p. 49). As always, his scholarship is excellent, but I am also not certain it is necessary to credit this charm to Peter, especially since his name is absent. If his name is indeed ubiquitous, then rendering it in Latin, even for someone whose Latin was poor, would not be particularly complicated. If Peter's name is absent, then perhaps we need not add in this patriarchal element to the charm, one that already addresses the ultimate patriarch.

59 M. L. Cameron, *Anglo-Saxon Medicine* (Cambridge: Cambridge University Press, 1993), p. 182. Brown rightly critiques their decision to group this with the *gefedan* remedies discussed above, and their choice to identify them all together as 'Pagan Rites for Miscarriage'. He notes: 'Grattan and Singer's solution of putting it with the three charms on fol. 185r–v, four pages on, is surely unwise, since each of those charms has its own heading and at least one of them, the third, is not about pregnancy but lactation, which would make this heading for child-bearing inappropriate. It seems simplest, therefore, to take this heading with the following words of the charm, as they stand.' Brown, 'Solving the "Solve" Riddle', p. 48.

60 Many thanks to Claire Taylor Jones for her assistance with this translation. In personal correspondence, she suggests that *catenis* is a dative noun, and notes the missing accusative, pointing out that we remain uncertain about 'whom or what is being released'. I was happy later

to see that Niles and D'Aronco translate this phrase as 'If a woman cannot give birth to a child. "God, command release from chains", three times'; *Anglo-Saxon Medical Texts*, Vol. I, p. 509.
61 Grendon 'Anglo-Saxon Charms', p. 162.
62 For conception, see Niles and D'Aronco, *Anglo-Saxon Medical Texts*, Vol. I, as follows: *OEM*, p. 380 (3.17); *OEH*, p. 234 (104.2); *OEM*, pp. 386 (5.12), 388 (5.13), 388 (5.14) – the latter for conception of a boy or a girl specifically.
63 The *Lacnunga* remedies for leaping over the grave, selling black wool and spitting milk.
64 *Lacnunga*'s Latin incantation; *OEH*, in Niles and D'Aronco, *Anglo-Saxon Medical Texts*, Vol. I, pp. 196 (82.1), 234 (104.2), 292 (143.3); and *LBIII*, in Cockayne, *Leechdoms*, Vol. II, p. 328 and 330 (37.1, 37.2).

4

Purging as treatment for miscarriage, stillbirth and conception

At stake in this chapter, and the subject of its final section, is the idea that women were not only responsible for but were also trusted with the identification of their own reproductive status, a privilege that is absent in much contemporary conversation about pregnancy and childbearing. Our ability to measure and track pregnancy via medical tools now often delimits the freedoms of women to control their own reproductive status and destiny. In certain cases, these tools present terrible dangers to contemporary people, rather than protecting them. Such was true for a Polish woman, identified to the public only as Izabela, who died in November 2021 in devoutly Catholic Poland as a result of the near total ban on the termination of pregnancy. At twenty-two weeks pregnant, she 'died of septic shock after doctors waited for her unborn baby's heart to stop beating'.[1] Despite scans indicating a range of defects, and the breaking of her amniotic sac at twenty-two weeks, the law's refusal to allow abortion if the foetus has a heartbeat prevented doctors from performing a procedure that would have saved this woman's life. In a text to her mother, she said 'thanks to the abortion law, I have to lie down. And there is nothing they can do. They'll wait until it dies or something begins, and if not, I can expect sepsis.' In such a case, the ability to perceive heartbeat interrupted the woman's own ability to identify what was happening inside her body, and to make a choice for her own health and safety.

Similarly, a law set forth in Texas in the autumn of 2021 not only intervenes in women's medical decisions, it encourages private citizens to report patients and physicians they believe to have terminated pregnancies, not only removing reporting from pregnant people themselves, but placing the ability to distinguish abortion from miscarriage in the hands of outsiders who might have little knowledge of the medical situation. Texas Senate Bill 8, which bans abortions after six weeks of pregnancy, also makes a proviso that 'private citizens can earn at least $10,000 for successfully reporting anyone who violated the law'.[2] In this case, private reporting is particularly dangerous as people may be persecuted for experiencing or treating miscarriages: 'If there are embryonic abnormalities that make the pregnancy non-viable but there is still cardiac activity', then the doctor performing the procedure can be sued.[3] While the law makes provisos about danger to the pregnant person's life, 'Doctors who decide to perform the procedure under these circumstances will have to determine how confident they are that the courts will agree with their opinion about whether those risks were present.'[4] Neither women nor their physicians are the primary arbiters of medical choice under this law, and the potential danger to a woman's life, as with Izabela, becomes a reality in Texas as well. Laws like these suggest that reproduction is a simple system, wherein a heartbeat at six weeks constitutes personhood, a belief that is not universally held.[5]

While contemporary medicine has the capacity to protect and support women's health, evangelical and conservative political and ideological beliefs use these same medical tools to intervene in women's medical decisions. The reliance of these laws on the mechanisms of heartbeat (present) and timing (six weeks) identify concrete limits that do not and cannot take into account medical complexity, leaving both women and their doctors in precarious medical and legal positions. In short: advances in reproductive medicine work to save women's lives, but also can be used to endanger them. Medieval women were not inhibited by such technological interventions. The tools to save people's lives, like Caesarian sections, might not have been available to early medieval women, but the lack of certain kinds of medical measurements and therefore a different focus on women's expertise over their own bodies offered a far less restrictive system than much of what is currently at work in Europe and the United States.

The medieval period is often held up as a time of conservative beliefs and practices that constrained women's lives. However, conservative contemporary beliefs about the reproductive process are in some ways far more draconian than medieval ones. What we now understand and believe about conception, pregnancy, miscarriage and abortion functions in very different ways than the beliefs we find embedded in early medieval English remedies. In fact, the lines between pregnant and unpregnant are far blurrier than we might imagine in a number of ways, opening up a space for a woman indeed to be an expert in her own body, and to select medical interventions to achieve personal outcomes. For instance, conception was understood to be a longer and more drawn out process, and consequently engaging in a practice to bring on menstruation or to purge tissue from the body would not necessarily be understood as abortive. Similarly, without contemporary medical mechanisms to measure, assess and track the development of the foetus, early medieval treatment for a late miscarriage would have relied on the word of the woman about how she perceived the state of a foetus.

I argue that in early medieval English medical texts, the division between remedies for stillbirth, miscarriage, abortion and purging is far less discrete than it is for us in western, culturally Christian societies of the twenty-first century. Treatments for purging seem to have included a range of causes including miscarriage and stillbirth, but also the removal of reproductive tissues generally, perhaps including the restoration of menses. I suggest that this facet of purging is not a method of validating, or figuratively naming, abortion, but rather offers a reframing of the idea, wherein that reproductive need is set parallel to the medical needs for intervention with miscarriage and stillbirth. In this sense, I argue not for a need for specificity and division, but rather for the value of a common category.

The range of terms used to describe purging, while discrete in certain ways, ultimately occupy the same conceptual space. First, I discuss the subset of these remedies that explicitly treat miscarriage and stillbirth, using variations of the phrase *deadboren tudor* ('dead-born offspring') to indicate what was being purged from the womb. These remedies indicate their function via the noun *tudor*, rather than with verbs like *clænsian* or *afeormian*, to indicate their purgative purpose. However, there are a range of other remedies for purging that shift focus from the noun (what is being purged) to the verb (purging itself). Such remedies reveal little information about what is being purged, or even why purging is required. Instead, the verbs *clænsian* and, more regularly, *afeormian* indicate the purging of tissue akin, but not identical, to the tissue expelled in miscarriage. While we might be tempted to understand those remedies for *clænsian* as affiliated with ritual impurity, I uncouple the notion of ritual cleansing from medical cleansing through an exploration of the term *clænsian*. Ultimately, I argue that remedies for both *clænsian* and *afeormian* function as purgative, both distinct from but also fundamentally related to those practices addressing the problem of miscarriage. Finally, I turn to a discussion of ensoulment in order to contextualise early medieval beliefs about reproductive timing, and the authority of women over their own bodies. Early medieval remedies understood pregnancy and conception in ways that are ulterior to contemporary understandings, and so current language struggles to encapsulate the medieval conception of these ideas.

Treating miscarriage and stillbirth: When a *tudor* is not a *cild*

Remedies for purging, including those for miscarriage and stillbirth, make up the second largest category of medical remedies for women in the early medieval English tradition, only outnumbered by remedies for menstrual woes, some of which seek similar outcomes as remedies for purgation. The volume of remedies for purging testifies to the known and understood dangers for reproductive women. Miscarriage and stillbirth were significant concerns for early medieval women, as is evident from the percentage of remedies specific to these maladies. In the case of both miscarriage and stillbirth, the only remedy is the safe removal of tissue that otherwise might lead to infection for the mother. These remedies therefore must be purgative in nature, and yet rarely use language that occurs elsewhere in the larger category of purging remedies (for example, the verbs *clænsian* or *afeormian*) to describe their purpose. Instead, they signify the idea of tissue in need of removal through the noun *tudor*. While these variations in language have been treated as interchangeable and may appear haphazard, in fact they reveal small but meaningful distinctions. In other words, while all of these remedies for purging seek to evacuate tissue, the causes for this need vary, and language is the means by which the cause is signalled. *Tudor* (offspring) and *cild* (child) may both signify remedies for miscarriage, but the former term widens the category of that which is to be purged, making space for a broader semantic notion of the work purging might do.

Miscarriage has been a common experience, both in the early Middle Ages and now. In both historical moments, treatments for miscarriage focus on restoring the mother's health (as opposed to preserving the pregnancy), although the methods by which they do so may be very different. Miscarriage occurs at a shockingly high rate, even in contemporary America under the best of circumstances; in fact, somewhere 'between one half and 96% of human conceptions end in early miscarriage'.[6] Later miscarriages are far rarer, with the risk dropping to approximately 3 per cent after twelve weeks and 0.6 per cent after twenty weeks.[7] While many miscarriages occur as a result of genetic abnormalities in the foetus, women's lived conditions also impact their ability to maintain a pregnancy. Medieval women were chronically undernourished, which affected their ability to become and remain pregnant, and so medieval rates for later miscarriages were likely much higher, as well as rates of stillbirth.[8] The only surprise about remedies for miscarriage in the Old English tradition is that there are not more of them. Those that do exist are for urgent medical needs: what happens when a woman's pregnancy does not continue to the birth of a living child? What happens when a child has died *in utero*? When a woman goes into labour far too early? In contemporary culture, medical professionals carefully monitor women, using ultrasounds to determine if a miscarriage is complete and if the uterus is empty. Miscarriages that take place later in a pregnancy are very likely to require an intervention like a dilatation and curettage (D&C), which requires the ability to open the cervix and remove any pregnancy tissue that remains.[9] Failing to remove pregnancy tissues can lead to infection because of the presence of bacteria, which can lead to septic shock and organ failure.[10] Infection and sepsis are also life-threatening to women after the birth of healthy children. Anna Wald notes that 'Maternal sepsis contributes substantially to maternal mortality, even in resource-rich countries.'[11] If these dangers exist even in the sophisticated medical system of the twenty-first century, then we can only presume that infection after miscarriage and childbirth were likely widespread and extremely dangerous in the early Middle Ages. Miscarriage and stillbirth must have been a significant concern for women.

The majority of language around miscarriage and stillbirth in early medieval medical remedies is fairly consistent, and focuses on the removal of a dead foetus. The remedies offer solutions for a *dead bearn* or *deadboren tuddor* ('dead child' or 'dead-born offspring'). This phrase, or variations of it, occurs eight times across the medical texts. Surprisingly, the word *dead* occurs only sixty times across the remedies, and refers most frequently to *deadspringas*, which are ulcers or carbuncles, although sometimes it refers to decaying flesh, or the deadly nature of an ingredient, and rarely if ever to the result of illness. In the gynaecological remedies, *dead* clarifies that a miscarriage has occurred, and that the foetus inside the woman is no longer alive. Although some remedies use language like *bearn* or *cild* (child, in both cases), most frequently the noun linked with *deadboren* is *tudor*. The term *tudor* occurs widely across the Old English corpus, including four times in the medical texts, consistently referring to miscarriage or stillbirth. Although the term carries general reference to 'offspring' elsewhere in the corpus, in the medical texts, it is directly associated with a foetus and, more specifically, with a non-viable foetus.[12] In other words, whenever we see this term in the medical texts, it refers not to a living baby, but to foetal tissue that needs to be removed.

In some remedies, the only clue as to what the remedy really does comes from this formulaic language. This is particularly true in remedies from the *OEM*, which uses animal ingredients, often strange ones, rather than herbal ingredients with known properties. For instance, the remedy using wolf's milk offers no clear indication of the result of the remedy, but tells us it is for a woman with a dead child inside her: 'Se wifman se þe hæbbe dead bearn on innoðe: gif he drinceð wylfene meolc mid wine and hunige gemenged gelice efne, sona hyt hælð' ('The woman who has a dead child inside her: if she drinks she-wolf's milk with wine and honey mixed together in the same quantity, it will immediately heal').[13] Despite the strangeness of the ingredient, the medical concern is expressed in clear terms: the woman retains a dead foetus inside her body. The remedy will result in quick healing, but there is no indication of how this healing operates. The solution seems to be almost entirely unclear – even the neuter pronoun 'hyt' disrupts meaning. Will the woman be healed? The dead child? What constitutes healing? Does this remedy offer resolution of the pregnancy in expulsion of the dead child? Perhaps this strange description of the result suggests an author uncertain of, or perhaps merely uninvested in, the remedy he transcribes. But perhaps this general reference to healing is exactly the kind of language people used for reproductive maladies that did not result in a living child: what is important is the problem (a dead-born child) and the final result (a healed maternal body). Naming purgation as the desired result given these circumstances may not have been necessary.

However, in both the *OEH* and *LBIII*, the pairing of the word *deadboren* with a commonly known emmenagogic and abortifacient ingredient, pennyroyal, makes clear the function of the remedy. Pennyroyal is well known as an abortifacient, and has been used for millennia across cultures. An abortifacient, in simple terms, is a substance that terminates a pregnancy by removing an embryo or foetus; an emmenagogue is a herb used to stimulate bloodflow and menstruation; many ingredients have both abortifacient and emmenagogic properties, and so the boundaries between the two may be blurry. John Riddle argues that the term emmenagogue offers a more socially acceptable title to herbs that fundamentally work as abortifacients; there is clear overlap between these categories.[14] When a woman has miscarried, she requires an abortifacient: she needs to terminate the pregnancy by expelling the foetus. Although pennyroyal has been used to end pregnancies or euphemistically 'bring on menstruation', it also causes uterine contractions, and even today shows up in conversations in pregnancy forums about inducing healthy labour naturally. The language in *OEH* makes clear that this latter goal does not apply, as it begins with the language of the 'dead-born child': 'Gyf deadboren cild sy on wifes innoðe: genim þysse ylcan wyrte þry cyþas, ond þa syn niwe swa hy swyþost stincen; cnuca on ealdon wine; syle drincan' ('If a stillborn child is in a woman's womb: take three sprigs of this same herb, and they should be so new that they smell most strongly; pound them in aged wine; give to drink').[15] *LBIII* uses a similar formulation both in terms of language and treatment, suggesting: 'Gif on wife sie deadbearn wyl on meolce and on wætre hleomoc and polleian sele drincan on dæg tuwa' ('If there is a dead child in a woman: boil brooklime and pennyroyal in milk and in water, give to drink twice a day').[16] Both remedies identify the problem in a passive and subjunctive structure – if a dead-born child *might be* inside a woman: she has not miscarried, but rather, a dead foetus exists inside her. The problem implicit in the existence of the 'dead-born child' is obvious: it must be expelled. Pennyroyal performs precisely this function, and thus the language for the malady and the herbal response make clear the outcome of the remedy without the necessity of an explicit description.

Dittany too is used for the treatment of stillbirth, but the remedy for stillbirth using dittany in the *OEH* also makes space for alternative uses, while clearly indicating the desired outcome. Like the pennyroyal remedy, the dittany remedy uses the familiar phrase for the malady (*deadboren tudor*) paired with a known abortifacient ingredient, but, even further, includes an explicit description of the result of consuming this herbal concoction:

> Gyf hwylc wif hæbbe on hyre innoðe deadboren tuddur genim þysse wyrte wos þe we dictamnum nemdun, gif heo butan fefere sy syle drincan on wine; gif hyre þone fefer derige, syle drincan on wearmum wætere. Sona hit þæt tuddur ut asendeþ butan frecnysse.
>
> [If a woman has a dead-borne fetus in her womb, take the juice of the herb we call dictamnus; if she does not have a fever, give it to drink in wine. If she suffers from fever, give it to drink in warm water. Immediately it will send out the fetus without danger.][17]

This remedy is remarkable and unique in its discussion of fever, a common indicator of infection and sepsis, a known danger for pregnant women and for those experiencing stillbirth or miscarriage. Further, its assurances of safety for the woman here are well founded: unlike pennyroyal, especially in oil form, dittany is relatively non-toxic in small amounts. But even more striking is its clear discussion of the result of the remedy: the 'sending out' of the foetus, identified early in the remedy as being already dead, but at the end lacking the adjective. This missing adjective, *deadboren*, might implicitly suggest uses beyond stillbirth for the removal of tissue, particularly given the attested history of the medical use of dittany.

In fact, dittany has been used to treat a range of reproductive ailments, depending on preparation and proportion. Ashley Buchanan explains that 'for more than 2,000 years, dittany was used as an emmenagogue: a substance to provoke menstruation', noting too its use in responding to 'delayed menstruation', about which she further clarifies 'delayed or missed menstruation in the early modern world could have been caused by any number of health and environmental factors. Pregnancy, however, was and remains a leading cause.'[18] This strong connection with resuming menstruation suggests a kind of continuum in terms of medical treatment for women's maladies. An ingredient that might simply return delayed menses, then in different proportions, or perhaps even the same ones, works to 'send out' a dead foetus, or even, perhaps, to cause an abortion (for example, sending out a *tuddor* that cannot be understood as *deadboren*). In this remedy, the outcome is clear and fixed, but the language leaves open space for the other kinds of work this ingredient might do via its purgative function.

While the use of dittany in this remedy opens up the possibility of application beyond stillbirth, the *OEH* remedy for wallflower actively combines the restoration of menstruation with the expulsion of foetal tissue. This remedy, unlike most others, identifies its primary purpose as menstrual – stirring the monthly courses – but states its function as both emmenagogic and abortifacient:

> Wyþ ða monoðlican to astyrigenne: genim þysse ylcan wyrte sædes, tyn penega gewihte on wine gecnucud ond gedruncen, oððe mid hunige gecnucud ond to ðam gecyndelican lime geled. Hyt þa monoðlican astyreþ ond þæt tudder of þam cwiðan gelædeþ.
>
> [To stir up menstruation: take ten pennies' weight of the seeds of this herb, pounded and drunk in wine, or mixed with honey and put on the genitals. It stirs up menstruation and leads out the fetus from the womb.][19]

In most cases, remedies state their general function at the start of a remedy: here, the desired goal is to stir up 'monoðlican', a regular monthly course. The remedy ends with a surprising – at least to contemporary readers – tag: that it will bestir menstruation *and* lead out foetal tissue from the reproductive organs. A contemporary reader might receive this remedy with shock – is this an abortion?! – but the remedy recounts it with no compunction. We might dwell on the connective word in the final line, 'and', asking if this remedy is meant to function this way only for women who wish to stir menstruation in this very specific way. But exploration of the ingredient does not offer an entirely satisfying answer, as wallflower historically has served a variety of reproductive purposes: 'The seeds in the form of a sitz bath or vaginal suppository have been administered as emmenagogue, abortifacient, and labor inducer',[20] depending on dosage. This remedy does not work to cover or occlude its language: it is clear about its goal and the method by which the goal is achieved.

It is tempting to read the remedy as an endorsement for abortion, but its work is more complex. Instead, it posits a reproductive cycle that operates differently than contemporary understandings of conception and pregnancy. It is important that the remedy uses the word *tudder*: the purgative effect of this herb is not to kill a child, but to purge tissue. The common but not constant affiliation of the word *tudder* with the phrase *deadboren* does not mean that all *tudder* are stillborn, but rather that a *deadboren tudder* is a specific kind of *tudder*, a foetus that has died late in pregnancy. But the focus of the wallflower's remedy on menstruation offers another understanding of *tudder*, as tissue from early pregnancy that can be purged in order to restore proper menstruation.

In certain ways, the problem for modern readers is one of contemporary colloquial language: we understand abortion and miscarriage as very different processes. However, in twenty-first-century medical language, miscarriage is identified as 'spontaneous abortion'. Daniela Blei notes that in other languages, like Spanish, the language for miscarriage and abortion is very close:

> Why use the separate word 'miscarriage', instead of the medical term, 'spontaneous abortion?' A British study says this separation is a recent phenomenon ... In Spanish, for example, one of my two mother tongues, it's either an 'abortion' or a 'spontaneous abortion'; there's no equivalent to miscarriage ... From a medical perspective, miscarriage and abortion are the same, even if the language we use and the emotions associated with the two experiences are not.[21]

Medically speaking, treatment for miscarriage and abortion (in certain conditions) are the same: the goal is the removal of tissue.

The difference is in the perception of this tissue; to use medieval terms, is it *cild* or is it *tudor*? The early medieval English medical manuscripts make this distinction in limited ways, which is not to say that they promote abortion.

Ingredients causing abortion were not unknown to medieval people, but the language for these practices and tools worked in different ways in order to package, and perhaps even to conceptualise, the processes of menstruation, miscarriage, conception, abortion and even birth. These early manuscripts manifest an alternative understanding of pregnancy, one that is dependent upon women to understand and advocate for their own bodies. The remedies for miscarriage and stillbirth suggest consistent emmenagogic and potentially abortifacient functions either explicitly or implicitly by virtue of their ingredients. Their goal is purgative: to remove something from inside a woman's body that she no longer wishes to have there. How medieval women might have thought about these experiences in certain ways necessarily differs from popular contemporary understandings. In early medieval England, not only miscarriages but stillbirths likely were frequent,[22] and there was little distinction between treating delayed menstruation and early pregnancy by means of emmenagogic and abortifacient ingredients. We cannot apply contemporary notions of what this medical treatment might have meant to the women who asked for or received it.

Clænsian: Ritual cleansing or medical cleansing?

While penitential texts affiliate women's bodies with ritual uncleanness, we find no evidence of this attitude in the medical texts. Not only are remedies that use the actual language of *clænsian* rare, they are concerned with the removal of unwanted tissue rather than the ritual cleansing of impure bodies. Particularly, given the menstrual laws discussed in Chapter 1, we know that ritual cleansing was a part of early medieval culture for women after giving birth and relative to menstrual cycles; medical *clænsian*, however, has little to do with this. Whereas, in religious texts, *clænsian* seems more closely aligned with the *DOE*'s second definition – 'to cleanse or purge of bodily impurity' (2.a) – in a more ritual sense, this is not so for the thirty or so remedies from the medical texts that make use of this same language, and which the *DOE* has linked under this definition.[23] There, the cleansing is not ritual at all; it is practical and medical.[24]

Impurity in the medical texts is not religiously ideological impurity, but rather literal uncleanness that can exacerbate illness. In fact, the medical texts' reasonably frequent use of this word often references the cleansing of wounds, as in a remedy in *Bald* treating liver trouble, which calls for an incision to be rinsed out regularly by means of a syringe: 'ac þu hie ælce dæge mid pipan geond spæt. 7 aþweah mid þam þingum siþþan oflege þe þa wunde clænsian' ('but each day you should rinse it through a tube, and wash it with that thing, afterwards, you should cover the wound to keep it clean').[25] The need for cleansing here is literal – to prevent infection; later the physician is urged to use honey for cleansing, should the wound become 'unsyfre' (impure).[26] Additionally, *clænsian* may invoke the idea of emptying out rather than cleaning of impurity. In *Bald*'s treatment for *wamb* disease (here, the *wamb* is described as 'fevered' when the man eats meat, so this is likely digestive), the sufferer is to undertake 'dægfæsten þæt mon mid þy þa wambe clænsige þæt hio þy þe leohtre sie' ('a day's fasting, so that with that he may cleanse the stomach so that it may be the lighter').[27] The *wamb*, or stomach, in this case is cleansed by means of being emptied. Therefore, while *clænsian* in the medical sense sometimes means cleaning away literal impurities and keeping a wound clean at the practical level, it also can mean 'emptying out'. I suggest that *clænsian* carries a wide semantic range, and so context is necessary to understand precisely the kind of cleansing that is at work. Some occurrences may carry meanings affiliated with figurative impurity, but in the medical texts, the impurities being treated by cleansing are more literal and concrete.

In fact, only one existing Old English remedy uses the word *clænsian* in reference to women's medicine, and it works as an intensifier for the remedy immediately previous to it for inducing menstruation. The first remedy in this pair, located in the *OEM*, and discussed more fully in Chapter 1, calls for the combing of a woman's hair then hanging hairs that come loose from a mulberry tree, and gathering them when they are 'clæne' (clean).[28] This idea continues two remedies later, and the author pushes on what this kind of cleansing might be:

> Gyf ðu wylle þæt wif sy geclænsod þe næfre mihte clene beon, wyrc hyre sealfe of þam feaxe, and hit æthwego adrig, & do on hyre lic, þonne byþ heo geclænsod.
>
> [If you wish to cleanse a woman who might never be clean, make her a salve with the hair, and let it dry a little, and put it on her body; then she will be cleansed.]²⁹

To provoke menstruation, loose hair must be ritually combed out and left to hang until clean, then gathered and preserved. But to cleanse a body, the hair must be gathered, hung and cleaned in the same way, and then must be worked into an unguent to be applied to the woman's body. In the first case, removing and hanging the hair promotes the removal of blocked menstruation: as hair is removed from the head, so might then whatever is understood to be preventing the woman's menstruation also be removed. The second case is more involved, and yet applies the same logic: the hair is removed, gathered and cleaned by virtue of tree-hanging, but then that cleaned item is reapplied to the body to initiate a cycle of more intensive cleansing. Mulberries, though not well attested in the early medieval textual tradition, have larger cultural affiliations with the purification of menstrual woes.³⁰ The Sephardic Jewish philosopher Maimonides indicates that 'the juice of the mulberry leaves in wine was a medicine for the bite of a venomous spider and against the "poison of menstrual blood"; alternatively, the mulberry root is used in Iran and Iraq "as a medicine against menstrual pains"'.³¹ Given the affiliation of the mulberry with menstrual afflictions, it seems likely that the second remedy, following closely after the first, and using the same ingredients, is meant to treat a similar malady. In the logic of the first case, a block is removed when the hair is removed and cleaned; in the second, the same result seems likely. And yet what cause might necessitate the levelling up of the remedy? This second remedy suggests it is for a woman 'þe næfre miht clene beon' ('who can never be clean'). Perpetual uncleanness could be a signal for ritual impurity, and yet there is no indication of this kind of impurity in the previous remedy. I suggest that the medical problem here is one that is more stubborn, rather than different. The next level of the remedy is meant as a shift not in the nature of the illness, but rather in its severity. In other words, whatever is blocking menstruation in the second case is more significant. If we consider the kinds of *clænsian* that occur in other remedies, the most likely method here is not cleaning an infected wound, but rather the act of emptying something out. In the case of gynaecological remedies, cleansing might well suggest the cleaning out of unwanted tissue.

Although *clænsian* occurs only in this one existing gynaecological remedy, it also appears in *Bald*'s 'Table of Contents' for gynaecological remedies (the remedies for which are lost), and its placement there helps denote the kinds of healing it does and does not convey. *Bald*'s list does not specify what *clænsian* means, but it does indicate what it does *not* mean. In other words, *Bald* gives an extensive list of gynaecological treatments that can indicate the discrete limits of each malady and treatment by virtue of contrast with others that are listed (I emphasise the relevant phrase below):

> Læcedomas wiþ wifa gecyndum forsetenum ond eallum wifa tydernessum: gif wif bearn ne mæge geberan, oþþe gif bearn weorþe dead on wifes innoþe, oððe gif hio cennan ne mæg, do on hire gyrdels þas gebedo swa on þisum læcebocum segþ.
>
> Ond manigfeald tacn þæt mon mæg ongitan hwæþer hit hyse cild þe mæden cild beon wille. Ond wiþ wifa adle. Ond gif wif migan ne mæge. *Ond gif wif ne mæge raðe beon geclænsod.*
>
> Ond wiþ wifa blodsihtan. Ond gif wif of gemyndum sie. Ond gif þu wille þæt wif cild hæbbe oþþe tife hwelp.
>
> Oþþe gif men cwið sie forweaxen, oþþe gif man semninga swigie, an ond feowertig cræfta.
>
> [Remedies for obstructed genitals of women and all infirmities of women: if a woman may not bear a child, or if a child becomes dead in a woman's womb, or if she may not give birth, put the prayer on her girdle just as this medical book says.
>
> And many signs that one may know whether it will be a boy child or a girl child. And for the disease of women. And if a woman cannot urinate. *And if a woman cannot be cleansed quickly.*[32]
>
> And for a haemorrhage of women. And if a woman might be out of her mind. And if you wish that a woman have a child, or a bitch, a pup.
>
> Or if the womb is distended in a person, or if one suddenly goes quiet, forty-one remedies.][33]

In this list, *Bald* offers remedies for obstructed genitals; for women who cannot give birth to a child; for women whose foetuses have died *in utero*; for determining the sex of an unborn child; for diseases of women generally; for women who cannot urinate; for women haemorrhaging, presumably after childbirth; for mental instability; for conception; for a distended womb; and even for women's silence. In the context of all of these other possible remedies, he specifically lists cleansing as its own discrete category. It is therefore distinct from conception, giving birth, haemorrhaging, urination, disease – all of the rest of the listed maladies. He suggests that the remedy in this category should be used 'gif wif ne mæge raðe beon geclænsod' ('if a woman cannot be cleansed quickly'). But why would cleansing be a time-sensitive matter? The timing indicated in the remedy is strange: for a woman who cannot be cleansed quickly. Does that mean 'quick' cleansing failed actually to clean her, and so she needs something more vigorous? Or does it mean she *urgently* requires cleansing? What kinds of women's reproductive maladies require this kind of haste? We know the remedy is not for childbirth, nor for a child who has died in the womb, nor for haemorrhage: the maladies that seem most in need of quick resolution. The other possibilities as I see it are the removal of a placenta, or the bringing on of an abortion or restoring the menstrual cycle prior to established and acceptable social time constraints. Therefore, although remedies for *clænsian* are rare, those that occur do not indicate a need for ritual cleansing for impurity; rather they function to remove unwanted tissue from the womb: they are intrinsically a part of the category of purging.

Afeormian: Treatment for early abortion as delayed menstruation

If we understand purging as a common category that uses a range of language for minor and often slippery variations, then we can use the more common verb *afeormian* to help understand in practical terms what *clænsian* might have meant. The *DOE* defines *afeormian* first as 'to clean, to free from impurity', with specific sections that feature the reproductive remedies 'of the body and its internal organs: to purge, purify'.[34] The notion of purification is attached to both cleaning and purging, which can help to explain the ways in which *clænsian* and *afeormian* might work as synonyms. And while the practice of 'cleaning' something might be an element present in both verbs, the medical remedies seem to focus most strongly on the removal of tissue by purging, rather than the notion of cleaning a wound. In the medical texts, the kinds of tissue to be expelled are specifically gynaecological. We might even wonder if these remedies could offer advice for childbirth. In fact, some remedies indicate that the same herbs are to be used for birth, listing different preparations and applications for the purposes of *afeormian*. These distinctions in use demonstrate first that purging works in similar ways to childbirth (i.e. these treatments are meant to 'get something out'), but birth and purging are clearly understood as requiring not only different treatment, but different language. I argue that remedies for purging specifically work to address that murky territory of early miscarriage/abortion/delayed menses, and that the Old English term *afeormian* invokes precisely this idea.

The herbs used for expelling foetal tissues are commonly also used for birth, although with different preparation and application. The *OEH* uses coniza (spikenard) both to aid in labour 'wið þæt wif cennan ne mæge' ('for that a woman cannot give birth'),[35] and to purge the womb: 'ðone cwiþan afeormaþ' ('purges the womb').[36] For birth, the woman is to lay a poultice on her genitals, whereas for cleansing purposes, she should sit on the poultice in order to achieve purging: 'on wætere gesoden 7 sittendum wife under geled heo ðone cwiþan afeormaþ' ('boiled in water and laid under a sitting woman, she will then purge her womb').[37] The distinctions between these remedies are small, and the similarities pronounced. Rather than laying the poultice directly on the genitals to induce labour, the same poultice is laid underneath the genitals of the woman while she is seated. We might presume, then, that the results of the two remedies are equally similar: to pull something out that doesn't want to come out, except that in one case what is to be brought forth is living, and in the other it is not. In fact, spikenard has been identified as a *partus preparator*, an ingredient used to prepare the pregnant body for birth. However, the safety and efficacy of this practice point to other potential uses for the same ingredient. Aviva Romm notes:

> Partus preparators are herbs used during the last weeks of pregnancy to tone and prepare the uterus for labor. Historically, they have been used to facilitate a rapid and easy delivery … The use of such herbs to prepare women for labor begs the question of why one would use an herbal preparation to prepare the body for something it naturally knows how to do. Furthermore, the safety of these herbs prior to the onset of labor is questionable.[38]

Romm suggests that the use of herbs like spikenard can be toxic to a foetus, and can result in miscarriage rather than contribute to a healthy delivery. Certainly the remedies for spikenard attempt to distinguish between the two uses: one for a woman who is ready to deliver her baby, and the other for a woman who wishes not to 'cennan' ('give birth'),[39] but rather to 'cwiþan afeormaþ' ('purge her womb').[40] The similarities between these treatments and the stated results suggest that this woman is looking not for purification, but rather to end (or perhaps to prevent, in the logic of beliefs of the time regarding conception) a non-viable pregnancy.

The *OEH* suggests the use of parsnip for a range of reproductive concerns for women, similarly demonstrating the distinction between categories of childbirth and purging. Parsnip's first listed use is for women giving birth 'earfuðlice', with difficulty, followed immediately by a remedy for purging. While the birthing remedy calls for the woman to bathe in the herbal solution, the purging remedy requires drinking, and uses the term *afeormian* in two different forms: 'Wið wifa afeormungæ: genim þas ylcan wyrte *pastinacam*; seoð on wætere, ond þonne heo gesoden beo, mengc hy wel ond syle drincan. Hy beoð afeormade' '(For purging of women, take this same herb, wild carrot, seethe it in water and, when it is boiled, mix it well and give it to drink. She will be purged').[41] The consistent proximity of purging remedies to those for childbirth suggests a parallel kind of gynaecological purgation; if this herb can help move along a difficult labour, its fundamental purpose is to help the body send out foreign elements. Indeed, it is known even today to promote uterine contractions. Contemporary research suggests that the chemical compound is dangerous for pregnant women to consume: 'Coumarin anti-coagulants are contraindicated in pregnant women because they cross the placenta and cause fetal bleeding in the uterus, increasing the probability of spontaneous abortion and fetal deformities.'[42] However, this research also indicates the historical use of the ingredient for menstrual purposes: 'Persian medicine believed that parsnip is an emmenagogue, so it was prohibited for pregnant women. Of course, this property has sometimes been used to treat amenorrhea or oligomenorrhea, which is today confirmed by the literature.'[43] This evidence suggests two things: first, the drug could cause spontaneous abortion/miscarriage, and second, discussing its use as relative to menstruation confirms the connection between delayed menstruation and abortion. The distinction in this formulation suggests that medieval medical practitioners knew what was at stake in the difference between these two uses. The fact that the parsnip is deployed topically for a woman in labour but is to be consumed by a woman in need of purging suggests a much more intense experience of the compound. In the case of the birthing woman, her body would have begun its own transition to labour, and so the herbs only needed to facilitate a process likely already under way. Also, the practitioner would need to be cautious about the impact of the herbs on the child being born. In contrast, purging would take place prior to the natural labour transitions of the birthing body, requiring stronger herbal induction, with no concern for the nature and safety of what is to be brought forth.

The term *afeormian* pushes beyond the typical language used to address menstruation, offering a positively framed term distinct from the language used for abortion. In contrast, penitential texts do not use *afeormian* to describe abortion or prohibited practices relative to pregnancy: they use other verbal formulations. For example, the *Scriftboc* relies on accreted verb phrases and verbs to indicate abortion, saying:

> Wif seo ðe *to æwyrpe gedo hire geeacnunga* in hire hrife ond *cwelle* ymbe xl nihta þæs ðe heo þam sæde onfo, ærðon hit gesawlad wære, swa se morðra, fæste iii winter ond æghwylcere wucan þa twegen dagas to æfenes ond ðreo æfesten. Gif hit *beorðer forleose*, i gear oððe iii æfesten.

> [A woman who *casts out the fetus* in her womb and *kills* it, if it is about 40 nights since she received the seeds, before it expired, she is, like the murderer, to fast 3 winters and every week is to keep the two fast days until evening and observe the three fasting periods. If she *loses the fetus*, she is to repent one year or the three fasting periods.][44]

The term *æwyrpan*, defined by the *DOE* as both 'casting out' and 'abortion', is used only once – here in the penitentials – to mean abortion. The *Thesaurus of Old English* lists two other terms for abortion – *awegaworpenness* (a variation of *æwyrpan*), and *beorþorcwelm* – the former appearing only once, also in the penitentials, and the latter, also only once, in the glossaries.[45] The penitential here goes to great lengths to clarify the result of the 'casting out', indicating not once but twice that such an act results in the death of the foetus.[46] The penitential also distinguishes between the killing of the foetus and 'losing' it. In the case of killing, the formerly pregnant person is treated as a murderer. In the case of losing, her penance is lighter, suggesting a range of responses to the termination of a pregnancy under different circumstances. In contrast to penitential texts, medical texts do not use the language of 'killing' to identify the work of purging; these practices are not understood as synonymous. In the medical texts, the verb *afeormian* adeptly indicates its contraceptive function because it uses existing language, language that can function medically as well as religiously (in the sense of purification) with positive connotations of removing something unwanted or even dangerous to the body that hosts it.

Perhaps even by identifying *afeormian* as a word indicative of what we now understand as abortion, we muddy the waters of thinking about the reproductive landscape of early medieval England. *Afeormian* might well be a treatment for (early) miscarriage as well as for abortion – but to an early medieval woman there might be very little difference between the two, both working as they do to facilitate the purging of tissue from the womb. As Riddle suggests,

> When women took menstrual regulators to stimulate the menses, they probably knew what it would do to a pregnancy. As we noted, the concept of pregnancy differs from our own. In the terms of the Middle Ages, a male seed was still in the body; in our terms, conception had taken place and was the reason for menstrual interruption.[47]

Riddle argues the that women took these herbs to manifest reproductive control, a claim that is countered by both Monica Green and Emily Kesling, who note that while the drugs do have this function, that does not mean that women regularly used them to cause abortion. However, more valuable in Riddle's claim is the medieval belief of conception as a continuum. This idea of that continuum is borne out by the actual real-life medical function of the herbs. A woman cannot engage in or be accused of killing her foetus if she is not yet pregnant. An abortifacient and an emmenagogue ideologically perform the same work in that they return a woman to her regular menstrual cycle, and if they do so by intervening in the drawn-out process of conception, then they do so by the process of purging, *afeormian*, not casting out, *æwyrpan*.

Both Green and Kesling dispute Riddle's claims about the use and availability of abortion, contesting his claims about textual transmission and biochemical means rather than about ideologies of pregnancy and conception. Green suggests: 'There is, then, very little evidence that medieval women regularly had access to any of the written texts that Riddle cites', continuing 'My survey of the available literature for medieval Europe shows attempts to disrupt fertility, but undercuts Riddle's assumption that biochemical means were most relied on and that this knowledge was primarily the property of women. True, we do find occasional statements about "womanly arts" of limiting fertility.'[48] Green's argument – that women likely had little access to medical texts, and that their ability to make use of the ingredients in the correct dosages was limited – are valid critiques of the practical nature of this problem. The existence of a textual tradition, as always, has a complicated relation with the actual people it purports to serve. Green reminds us that in an illiterate culture, the passing down of such information would be challenging at best, and the skills to produce and apply remedies limited:

> The actual ability to use fertility-enhancing or -disrupting herbs depends on close knowledge of soils, harvesting times, preparation methods, administration doses, et cetera. For such knowledge to be sustained in an illiterate society would depend on uninterrupted continuation of the practices that generated the knowledge in the first place. Thus, even if (in raw chemical terms) an emmenagogue can be 'flipped' to become an abortifacient, effective use of such a substance in this way would entail the continuation of practices by communities that used the technology often enough to keep the knowledge alive.[49]

So many of the ingredients and preparations included in this chapter and this book might have been largely inaccessible to early medieval English women. Where wolf's milk is a magical ingredient neither reasonably procured nor even desirable, finding a non-native mulberry tree might prove just as difficult. Even with familiar and accessible ingredients like pennyroyal, determining the correct proportions and preparations might be beyond the scope of ordinary women. And yet, women across cultures and epochs have gone and will go to extreme lengths not to have children. There is no reason to presume that these remedies for purging, whether or not they were actually usable – remedies that specifically result in the idea of exiting something from the womb of a woman – would not be intended to prevent conception, pregnancy or live births.

The early medieval boundaries around menstruation, conception, pregnancy, miscarriage and abortion are fluid in a way that often makes them difficult to discuss or pin down. Even Riddle, who argues for an expanded timeline for conception in order to complicate the question of abortion, falls back on the idea that remedies and the language around them work figuratively: 'As a rule, medieval writings were more reluctant to specify abortifacients than were classical works; instead they relied more on circumlocutions, such as menstrual stimulators.'[50] Emily Kesling gently pushes against Riddle's conflation of abortifacient and emmenagogue, noting that:

> John Riddle has argued that emmenagogues may have been frequently used in the ancient world and Middle Ages as abortifacients. If the translator of the *Herbarium* was aware of this, this might help explain why some of these types of remedies were omitted. However, more typically emmenagogic remedies would have been used in the Middle Ages to promote fertility in accordance with the belief that menstruation was part of the process of bodily purification necessary for conception.[51]

Kesling suggests potential textual editing to exclude those remedies understood to induce abortion in the absence of such remedies from the *OEH*, but ultimately concludes that this is likely not the case as those remedies would not have been understood as abortion-causing. Here, the line between remedies that work as emmenagogues in order to bring on menstruation and to increase fertility, and those that would have worked to purge tissue, is of little medical consequence. There is a linguistic distinction between remedies that provoke flow (*astyrian monoðlican* ('stir menstruation') discussed in Chapter 1), and those that purge tissue (*afeormian* ('purge')). The variation in language tells us that there is a difference between these remedies, but the ways in which these causes are treated is understood, as I have shown, on a continuum, with purging requiring adjustments to the less aggressive treatments for stirring menstruation.

All scholars who work on this material must wrestle with the question of knowledge. Did women understand conception differently than we do now? Did they believe they were pregnant during what we consider very early pregnancy? Could they have even known, in most cases, that they were pregnant in those first weeks post conception? And if they did, would they have had access to experts, texts and ingredients in order to prevent conception or bring on abortion? To some degree, we can answer questions of access: they likely did not have access to texts or practitioners who could give them accurate and effective treatments to bring on abortion. But the texts that remain give us language that suggests an extended timeline for conception, the necessity that women understand and dictate the timing of their own menstrual cycles, and the means by which women might regulate their own fertility.

Conclusions: Ensoulment, timing and the authority of women

Timing, in all phases of reproduction, is a crucial element, because of the fundamentally temporary nature of all elements of reproduction, but also because of the desire to anticipate and prepare. Relative to menstruation, young women wait to experience their first menstrual period, and then women live lives often dictated by their regular (or not) calendar of menstruation. When might a period begin? When will it end? What if it is late? Early? Absent? Pregnancy impinges on the timing of menstruation, connected inherently (in most pregnancies) by its absence. A woman comes to know she is pregnant because her period does not begin when it ought to. Pregnancy continues along this new trajectory of timing, a countdown to childbirth. In contemporary measures in the USA, we count to forty weeks. That timing is, of course, absurd in many ways. In this calendar of forty weeks, a woman is considered pregnant before conception actually occurs: that counting begins with the end of a woman's last menstrual period. And so the timing attempts to account for something internal that is often difficult to pinpoint. When, exactly, does conception occur? In contemporary terms, we want to know so that medical assessments and tests and due dates can be calculated, and all outcomes managed as much as possible. This was certainly true for medieval women as well – determining when a baby might arrive was certainly a familiar calculation, as we can see in the passage discussed in Chapter 2 concerning the development of the foetus. But that passage also points to another reason to determine the moment of conception, and it has to do with the development of the soul. There, the author of the prognostic on the development of the foetus indicates that in the third month 'he biþ man butan sawle' ('he is a man without a soul').[52] Indeed, the prognostic does not tell us when he *does* develop this soul, but remarks only upon its absence. Perhaps, in fact, it is the absence that is most important, when thinking about foetal development, particularly in a time with precarious pregnancy outcomes.

Ensoulment marks the moment in which a conceived foetus develops a soul. Badawy Khitamy notes the debate in early western Christianity between notions of immediate and delayed ensoulment. He clarifies: 'The delayed ensoulment theory dates back to the time of Aristotle, who argued that ensoulment for males is 40 days and 90 days for females.'[53] He notes that this demarcation exists across traditions and cultures:

> The Qur'an and the tradition of the Prophet Muhammad declared the ensoulment period to be about 120 days (4 lunar months plus 10 days) computed from the moment of conception, which is equivalent to 19 weeks and one day, or 134 days from a woman's last menstrual period. Prior to this period, the human embryo has sanctity which gradually increases with its development. It is considered as a person after ensoulment.[54]

Thus ensoulment marks a threshold for determining humanity, one that is complicated to determine, and for which a range of metrics and disagreements have arisen across and within religious and ethical traditions.[55] To suggest that ensoulment is simple and clear would be disingenuous, but to argue that a foetus in the early stages of pregnancy was treated in exactly the same way as a foetus in the later stages would be untrue.

One of the particular complications around ensoulment has to do with the measuring of pregnancy and pinpointing conception. This calculation depends on accurate memory and reporting, and an accurate sense, even, of the passage of time for people who had little ability or need to record mundane occurrences – like a monthly period. This is not to suggest a lack of awareness of the body for early medieval women, but rather, given the likely irregularity of menstruation and the absence of personal calendars, that the accurate counting of such time might have been complicated and difficult. Many women claim to know the moment they conceive, but this is not a universal truth: in fact, determining pregnancy without contemporary medical tools is difficult in the early stages, even for highly educated experts. In an interview, currently practising midwife Melinda Rodriquez-Salus says:

> At six weeks of pregnancy (about forty-two days) the baby is about ¼ to ½ inch and 1/1000 of an ounce. The unpregnant uterus is the size of a plum. At six weeks a woman likely won't know she is pregnant and her uterus is the size of an apple but still sitting below the pelvis. Basically it would all be guesswork until the uterus rose above the pelvis at about twelve weeks … twice the number of days after ensoulment. There would have been NO medical way to tell if she was absolutely pregnant at seven weeks of pregnancy.[56]

The physical markers of early pregnancy are largely unreadable and uncertain, and so any legal or penitential system relying on the accurate counting of time would be ineffective, in actual practice. Therefore, these parameters for ensoulment are academic and intellectual markers that are fundamentally unusable by the population at large.

As with so many of the prescriptions and prohibitions regarding women's reproductive behaviour, the notion of ensoulment is an attempt to place arbitrary and measurable limits on bodies incongruent with those units of measure. Establishing and promoting notions of ensoulment, and building those into penitential models for infant loss, are attempts to police pregnant bodies, much like the current heartbeat laws that endanger women's lives today. Who could tell whether the loss of a pregnancy was the result of abortion or miscarriage? In his discussion of remedies for stillbirth, Riddle clarifies that women were the arbiters of their own pregnancy status:

Many of the classical texts and some medieval ones said only that the drugs expelled a dead fetus. A woman who declared her fetus dead, as best we can tell, would have her word accepted. Thus a physician who assisted her would not knowingly deliver an abortion. He would believe that he was engaging in a therapeutic act. Neither the physician nor others in the household or community would know that what killed the fetus was the drug that was taken to expel a dead fetus. Medieval society was similar to ancient Greek society in the way it regarded a woman's word as being the determinant of pregnancy.[57]

Women's word regarding their pregnancy or the loss of that pregnancy was in most cases the only word that mattered. Given the difficulty of determining pregnancy for a woman at this time, and given the nutritional climate in which women lived, would a woman even know for sure the status of her own pregnancy, or if the foetus inside her was dead or alive? Might a woman experiencing a miscarriage fear that she had done something to hurt her foetus, even unwittingly? The lines between abortion and miscarriage seem finer than the contemporary language for these categories ascribes, where Old English offers some space around and within its own named categories. It is the woman, then, who must make sense of her own physical experiences, and decide what it is she has suffered and what kinds of help, physical or spiritual, that she requires. The systems embedded in the penitentials, like those regarding the timeline related to ensoulment, can work in a variety of ways. In part, they embed a set of values regarding pregnancy (i.e. it is wrong to abort a foetus, but it's more wrong to abort one that has developed a soul), but they also work to make space for the kind of uncertainty that is attached to pregnancy and infant loss.[58]

Is it better or worse to live in a time with technologies that *can* help women, but with practitioners who may refuse to do so? Religious conservatives frequently situate their own repression of women's reproductive choices in what they perceive as originary or early Christian ethics. But the early medieval English medical texts show us a far more nuanced and complex narrative relative to women's bodies and reproductive practices. We might scoff at remedies that suggest wolf's milk can help a woman expel her stillborn baby, or that combing one's hair and hanging it from a mulberry tree can work as a purgative agent. But these remedies demonstrate a practice of listening to and believing women when they ask for medical assistance. Alas, for women in Texas, and for women like Izabela in Poland, the advanced medicine of our contemporary moment does not grant them the same authority over their own bodies and medical needs. Make no mistake: being a woman of reproductive age in early medieval England was profoundly dangerous, and the medical tradition could do little to help women with exigent gynaecological needs.

It is no surprise that early medieval English women might have wanted to control their fertility, and used a variety of methods to increase and decrease fertility. What is surprising is the linguistic sophistication of Old English that works to distinguish with nuance the categories of treatment and need relative to pregnancy, conception and foetal loss. While the remedies for purging uniformly work to remove tissue from women's reproductive organs, they offer a range of language to describe this process, focusing alternatively on what is expelled (*deadboren tudor*) or on the process of purging (*clænsian* and *afeormian*). They do not use the language of legal or penitential infanticide or abortion, nor do they identify women's bodies as abject or taboo. These remedies give us the imagined voices of women asking to be purged of tissue that might endanger their lives in a number of ways: whether women had access to these specific remedies is immaterial. The request and the response in these medical texts demonstrate a belief in women, and their ability to identify their own reproductive status and needs.

Notes

1 Anna Włodarczak-Semczuk and Kacper Pempel, 'Death of Pregnant Woman Ignites Debate about Abortion Ban in Poland', Reuters (6 November 2021), www.reuters.com/world/europe/death-pregnant-woman-ignites-debate-about-abortion-ban-poland-2021-11-05/ (accessed 10 December 2021).
2 Julie Mazziotta, 'Texas Website where People Can Report Violators of Abortion Ban Shut Down a Second Time', *People* (7 September 2021), https://people.com/health/texas-site-to-report-violators-of-the-highly-restrictive-abortion-law-shut-down-a-second-time/ (accessed 10 December 2021).

3 Peter Holley and Dan Solomon, 'Your Questions about Texas's New Abortion Law, Answered', *Texas Monthly* (7 October 2021), www.texasmonthly.com/news-politics/texas-abortion-law-explained/ (accessed 10 December 2021).
4 Ibid.
5 Christina Han and Cara C. Heuser, 'Antiabortion Heartbeat Bills Are Neither Morally nor Legally Sound', *Scientific American* (23 January 2023), www.scientificamerican.com/article/antiabortion-heartbeat-bills-are-neither-morally-nor-legally-sound/ (accessed 15 July 2023). Pew Research suggests that 'nearly four-in-ten endorse the notion that "human life begins at conception, so a fetus is a person with right" (26% say this describes their views extremely well, 12% very well)', in Pew Research Center, 'America's Abortion Quandary' (6 May 2022), www.pewresearch.org/religion/2022/05/06/americas-abortion-quandary/ (accessed 15 July 2023). For more on contemporary abortion bans, see the sources cited in Chapter 2 n. 4. Despite being published prior to *Dobbs vs Jackson*, the following article offers a clear discussion of international social context of abortion in the early twenty-first century: Frances Raday and the Working Group on the issue of discrimination against women in law and in practice, 'Women's Autonomy, Equality and Reproductive Health in International Human Rights: Between Recognition, Backlash and Regressive Trends', *United Nations Human Rights Special Procedures* (October 2017), www.ohchr.org/WomensAutonomyEqualityReproductiveHealth.pdf (accessed 15 July 2023). See also PBS, 'How the U.S. Compares with the Rest of the World on Abortion Rights', *PBS News Hour* (1 July 2022), www.pbs.org/newshour/politics/how-the-u-s-compares-with-the-rest-of-the-world-on-abortion-rights (accessed 15 July 2023).
6 Scott Forbes, *A Natural History of Families* (Princeton: Princeton University Press, 2005), p. 81.
7 Krissi Danielsson, 'Making Sense of Miscarriage Statistics', *Verywell Family* (20 April 2020), www.verywellfamily.com/making-sense-of-miscarriage-statistics-2371721 (accessed 25 June 2021). Miscarriage and stillbirth are counted differently, as miscarriage is understood to occur prior to twenty weeks, and stillbirth after twenty weeks of pregnancy. The Center for Disease Control and Prevention data from 2020 say that about 21,000 stillbirths were reported, noting a significant improvement in reduction of stillbirth rates after 1940 as a result of better maternal care; Center for Disease Control and Prevention, 'Stillbirth: Data and Statistics' (last reviewed 4 October 2022), www.cdc.gov/ncbddd/stillbirth/data.html (accessed 16 July 2023). However, race disparities continue to affect certain groups disproportionately.

They note that 'in 2020, fetal mortality rates continued to vary by race and Hispanic origin; rates were highest for non-Hispanic NHOPI [Native Hawaiian or Other Pacific Islander] (10.59) and non-Hispanic Black (10.34) women, followed by non-Hispanic AIAN [American Indian or Alaska Native] (7.84) women'. Elizabeth C. W. Gregory, Claudia P. Valenzuela and Donna L. Hoyert, 'Fetal Mortality: United States, 2020', *National Vital Statistics Reports*, 71.4 (4 August 2022), 1–19 (p. 4).

8 Vern Bullough and Cameron Campbell note significant protein and iron deficiencies in the diet of early medieval peasants, particularly for menstruating, pregnant and lactating women, which likely contributed to negative reproductive consequences, in 'Female Longevity and Diet in the Middle Ages', *Speculum*, 55.2 (1980), 317–25 (p. 319). We know that 'iron is essential for placental and fetal development and severe iron deficiency can cause adverse pregnancy outcomes such as increased risk of preterm labor, fetal loss, and even perinatal death'; Yifan Guo, Na Zhang, Daoqiang Zhang et al., 'Iron Homeostasis in Pregnancy and Spontaneous Abortion', *American Journal of Hematology*, 94.2 (February 2019), 184–8, DOI: 10.1002/ajh.25341 (accessed 8 December 2021). Little archaeological evidence of miscarriage exists because this kind of tissue decomposes.

9 Approximately 50 per cent of reported miscarriages require this procedure; American Pregnancy Association, 'D&C Procedure after a Miscarriage', https://americanpregnancy.org/pregnancy-complications/d-and-c-procedure-after-miscarriage/#:~:text=A%20D%26C%2C%20also%20known%20as,the%20contents%20of%20the%20uterus (accessed 3 June 2020). This kind of treatment would have been unavailable to medieval women, as Sally Crawford notes that early medieval doctors 'eschewed surgery except of the most superficial type – given the high risk of infection at the time, any incision in the body would have been highly likely to lead to death'; Sally Crawford, *Childhood in Anglo-Saxon England* (Stroud: Sutton, 1999), p. 61.

10 Krissi Danelsson, 'Complications after a Miscarriage', *Verywell Family*, www.verywellfamily.com/possible-complications-after-a-miscarriage-2371525 (accessed 3 June 2020).

11 Anna Wald, 'Comment: When Postpartum Maternal Sepsis Is Fatal', *NEJM Journal Watch* (23 September 2019), www.jwatch.org/na49866/2019/09/23/when-postpartum-maternal-sepsis-fatal (accessed 3 June 2020), commenting on Matthew Hensley, Melissa E. Bauer, Lindsay K. Admon and Hallie C. Prescott, 'Incidence of

Maternal Sepsis and Sepsis-Related Maternal Deaths in the United States', *JAMA*, 322.890 (3 September 2019), DOI:10.1001/jama.2019.9818 (accessed 3 June 2020).

12 A search of the *DOE Web Corpus* shows that *tudor*, with its spelling variants, occurs 119 times, and means 'that which grows from another (used of animals or of plants), offspring, progeny, product, fruit'. Joseph Bosworth, 'túdor', in *An Anglo-Saxon Dictionary Online*, ed. Thomas Northcote Toller, Christ Sean and Ondřej Tichy (Prague: Faculty of Arts, Charles University, 2014), https://bosworthtoller.com/31117 (accessed 23 December 2023).

13 John P. Niles and Maria D'Aronco (eds and trans), *Anglo-Saxon Medical Texts*, Vol. I, *The Old English Herbal, Lacnunga, and Other Texts*, Dumbarton Oaks Medieval Library (Cambridge, MA: Harvard University Press, 2023), p. 406 (10.7).

14 John M. Riddle, *Contraception and Abortion from the Ancient World to the Renaissance* (Cambridge, MA: Harvard University Press, 1994), p. 270.

15 Niles and D'Aronco, *Anglo-Saxon Medical Texts*, Vol. I, p. 218 (94.6).

16 Thomas Oswald Cockayne, *Leechdoms, wortcunning, and starcraft of early England. Being a collection of documents, for the most part never before printed, illustrating the history of science in this country before the Norman Conquest*, 3 vols (London: Longman, Green, Longman, Roberts and Green, 1864–66), Vol. II, p. 330 (37.4).

17 Niles and D'Aronco, *Anglo-Saxon Medical Texts*, Vol. I, p. 168 (63.1).

18 The lack of measurement of any ingredients is a strange quality of these texts, particularly given the toxic nature of many of the suggested herbs. This lack of measurement might suggest that readers were well versed in appropriate measures and did not need guidance, but it also suggests that perhaps these remedy books were used not as recipes, but rather simply as references. Ashley Buchanan notes: 'Contemporary research on pennyroyal's key active compound, pulegone, has revealed that the plant's essential oil does have the potential to produce significant effects on the female reproductive system. But there is some danger involved: Pulegone also makes pennyroyal toxic, and plants in different regions and climates produce varying amounts of it, making proper dosage difficult.' Ashley Buchanan, 'Plant of the Month: Dittany', *JStor Daily* (23 September 2020), https://daily.jstor.org/plant-of-the-month-dittany/ (accessed 13 July 2021).

19 Niles and D'Aronco, *Anglo-Saxon Medical Texts*, Vol. I, p. 330 (165.4).
20 Ghazaleh Mosley, Parmis Badr, Amir Azadi, Zohreh Abolhassanzadeh, Seyed Vahid Hosseini and Abdolali Mohagheghzadeh, 'Wallflower (*Erysimum cheiri* (L.) Crantz) from Past to Future', *Research Journal of Pharmacognosy*, 6.2 (2019), 85–95 (p. 86).
21 Daniela Blei, 'The History of Talking about Miscarriage', *The Cut* (23 April 2018), www.thecut.com/2018/04/the-history-of-talking-about-miscarriage.html (accessed 2 December 2021).
22 It is difficult to obtain numerical data of stillbirths in the early Middle Ages because foetal remains are rarely well preserved, and even then only if they coincide with maternal mortality, although some stillbirth remains can be located in burials; see Madison Crow, Colleen Zori and Davide Zori, 'Doctrinal and Physical Marginality in Christian Death: The Burial of Unbaptized Infants in Medieval Italy', *Religions*, 11.12 (2020), 678. Giulia Riccomi, Cristina Felici and Valentina Giuffra state: 'In utero fetuses are rarely reported in the osteoarchaeological literature. In particular, first-trimester fetuses are seldom documented, as a low level of bone mineralization in this gestation phase prevents proper preservation and/or identification. Some evidence of second-trimester fetuses is available, but the majority of findings of fetal remains can be linked to the third trimester of gestation'. 'Maternal-Fetal Death in Medieval Pieve di Pava (Central Italy, 10th–12th Century AD)', *International Journal of Osteoarchaeology*, 31.5 (2021), 701–15 (pp. 701–2).
23 'Clænsian', in Angus Cameron, Ashley Crandell Amos, Antonette diPaolo Healey et al. (eds), *Dictionary of Old English: A to I Online* (Toronto: Dictionary of Old English Project, 2018), https://tapor.library.utoronto.ca/doe/ (accessed 23 December 2023), definition 2.a.
24 The *DOE* might well have fitted these occurrences under definition 1.a., 'to cleanse, free from dirt or filth', although the occurrences listed there also invoke a religious kind of cleansing, including citations from Bede, *Soul to Body*, and a homily. *Geclænsod* is a common enough word, but of its 102 occurrences in the corpus, the majority refer to a religious kind of cleansing, a ritual purification against sin. That resonance does not appear to exist in medical texts.
25 Cockayne, *Leechdoms*, Vol. II, pp. 208 and 210 (22.2.10).
26 Ibid., Vol. II, p. 210. *Unsyfre* is a relatively rare word, occurring only nine times in the corpus, and only once in the medical texts. It is used to identify 'impure speech' in *Confessionale Pseudo-Egberti*, header, 7.5, as cited in the *DOE Web Corpus*.
27 Cockayne, *Leechdoms*, Vol. II, pp. 216 and 218 (25.1).

28 Niles and D'Aronco, *Anglo-Saxon Medical Texts*, Vol. I, p. 374 (2.2). They translate this word as 'free from impurities' (p. 375).
29 Ibid., p. 374 (2.4).
30 Mulberry trees occur only eight times in the *DOE Web Corpus*, three of which are in *OEM*, and all but one beyond this occur in glosses, with one occurrence in Ælfric's Homily 12. Despite the rarity of the name, there is some evidence that they existed in London as early as the fifth century, brought by the Romans, and were grown in monasteries and abbeys; *Moris Londiniium*, 'Timeline of the Mulberry in London', www.moruslondinium.org/research/timeline (accessed 30 July 2021).
31 Efraim Lev and Zohar Amar, *Practical 'Materia Medica' of the Medieval Eastern Mediterranean According to the Cairo Genizah* (Leiden: Brill, 2008), p. 452.
32 *Geclænsod* is translated as 'purified' in Debby Banham and Christine Voth (eds and trans), *Old English Medicine in British Library, Royal D. xvii*, Vol. II of *Anglo-Saxon Medical Texts*, Dumbarton Oaks Medieval Library (Cambridge, MA: Harvard University Press, forthcoming). Cockayne translates it as 'cleansed'; *Leechdoms*, Vol. II, p. 173.
33 Cockayne, *Leechdoms*, Vol. II, p. 172 (60).
34 'Afeormian', in *DOE*, including 1.b.iii.
35 Niles and D'Aronco, *Anglo-Saxon Medical Texts*, Vol. I, p. 292 (143.3).
36 Ibid., p. 292 (143.2). They translate it as 'cleanses' (p. 293), while De Vriend translates this phrase as 'purifies the womb'; Hubert Jan De Vriend (ed.), *The Old English Herbarium and Medicina de Quadrupedibus*, Early English Text Society (Oxford: Oxford University Press, 1984), p. 354.
37 Niles and D'Aronco, *Anglo-Saxon Medical Texts*, Vol. I, p. 292 (143.2).
38 Aviva Romm, *Botanical Medicine for Women's Health* (London: Churchill/Livingstone, 2010), p. 325.
39 Liuzza, *Anglo-Saxon Prognostics: An Edition and Translation of Texts from London, British Library, MS Cotton Tiberius A.iii* (London: D. S. Brewer, 2011), p. 200.4.
40 Ibid., p. 292 (143.2).
41 Liuzza, *Anglo-Saxon Prognostics*, p. 200.4.
42 Hoorieh Mohammadi Kenari, Gholamreza Kordafshari, Maryam Moghimi, Fatemeh Eghbalian and Dariush Taher Khani, 'Review of Pharmacological Properties and Chemical Constituents of *Pastinaca sativa*', *Journal of Pharmacopuncture*, 24.1 (31 March 2021), 14–23 (p. 23).

43 Ibid.
44 Allen Frantzen (ed.), *Anglo-Saxon Penitentials: A Cultural Database*, Oxford, Bodleian Library, Junius 121, s. XI¾; Worcester, 93b. X14.07.01, www.anglo-saxon.net/penance/index.php?p=JUNIUS_93b (accessed 16 July 2023). *Æwyrp* occurs only three times in the *DOE Web Corpus*, twice in Benedict's Rule indicating a more literal casting out of people, and once, noted above, in the penitentials. The latter can be paralleled in the Latin form, 'abortivum', while the former uses the Latin 'ajiectio'.
45 Liuzza, *Anglo-Saxon Prognostics*, p. 200.6.
46 This repetition also suggests that a woman might need to repent if she *attempts* an abortion unsuccessfully, with different penitential requirements if she succeeds.
47 John M. Riddle, 'Contraception and Early Abortion in the Middle Ages', in Vern L. Bullough and James A. Brundage (eds), *Handbook of Medieval Sexuality* (New York: Garland, 1996), pp. 261–77 (p. 268).
48 Monica Green, 'Gendering the History of Women's Healthcare', *Gender & History*, 20.3 (2008), 487–518 (pp. 503, 505).
49 Ibid., p. 502.
50 Riddle, 'Contraception and Early Abortion', p. 270.
51 Emily Kesling, *Medical Texts in Anglo-Saxon Literary Culture* (Cambridge: D. S. Brewer, 2020), p. 201.
52 Liuzza, *Anglo-Saxon Prognostics*, p. 201.
53 Badaway A. B. Khitamy, 'Divergent Views on Abortion and the Period of Ensoulment', *Sultan Qaboos University Medical Journal*, 13.1 (February 2013), 26–31 (p. 28). D. A. Jones addresses more fully the difficulty of the critical tradition in determining early attitudes and their origin. He critiques an influential essay by G. R. Dunstan for an important omission: 'This unfortunate mistranslation had an extensive influence on later writers. Dunstan quotes a passage from Augustine to the effect that killing an unformed embryo is not homicide: If what is brought forth is unformed but at this stage some sort of living, shapeless thing, then the law of homicide would not apply, for it could not be said that there was a living soul in that body, for it lacks sense, if it be such as is not yet formed and therefore not yet endowed with sense [G. R. Dunstan, *The Artifice of Ethics* (London: SCM Press, 1974), p. 87]. Nevertheless, Augustine's attitude is more ambiguous than it might seem and this becomes evident if we examine this passage more closely. This is made difficult because, unaccountably and without warning the reader, Dunstan has deleted a whole line from the middle of the passage. After "living, shapeless thing" Augustine adds the qualification "since the great question of

the soul is not to be rushed into rashly with a thoughtless opinion". This raises the issue of the origin of the soul, a question which Augustine discusses in many of his writings. Augustine remained open to the view that the soul was generated by the parents, as this seemed to explain the inheritance of original sin. This view implies that the soul is present from conception. By deleting the line Dunstan conceals the fact that Augustine's account of the origin of soul is in tension with the rest of this passage.' D. A. Jones, 'The Human Embryo in the Christian Tradition: A Reconsideration', *Journal of Medical Ethics*, 31 (2005), 710–13 (p. 711).

54 Khitamy, 'Divergent Views', p. 29.
55 John Riddle notes the development of thinking regarding ensoulment from Aristotle's original observations about animation through Albert the Great's thirteenth-century claims that the embryo retained status only as an animal prior to receiving its soul, while St Thomas Aquinas and Giles of Rome, both in the thirteenth century, declared the soul to be made by God and not by human parents, and thus affirmed the animal nature of the embryo prior to ensoulment. Riddle, 'Contraception and Early Abortion', pp. 266–7.
56 In an interview with the author, 5 March 2020.
57 Riddle, 'Contraception and Early Abortion', p. 271.
58 Various opinions regarding contraceptive and abortive practices in Islam exist. Abortion with no medical reasons might be considered a crime in Islam, and 'the degree of crime', affirmed Imam Ghazali, 'increases from phase to phase. The first stage is when the sperm in the uterus mixes with the woman's fluid (ova) and becomes ready to receive life. Destroying it (i.e. the zygote) is a crime. The crime becomes more serious when aborting the alaqa or mudh'gha (clot). The degree of crime becomes even more serious when aborting the fetus after ensoulment or before its birth (as it is considered homicide)'; Khitamy, 'Divergent Views', p. 29. However, Basim F. Musallam argues that once the contraceptive practice of '*azl* (withdrawal) was allowed, this opened wide a range of contraceptive and abortive practices'; *Sex and Society in Islam* (Cambridge: Cambridge University Press, 1983). As a review of the book by G. H. A. Juynboll states, '*every* possible and impossible means of birth control, *including* abortion, became perfectly permissible and widely resorted to, if we go by the extensive lists of contraceptive recipes enumerated in this book … In other words, twentieth-century birth control discussions do not constitute a logical continuation of an age-old dispute in Islam between "decent" and "indecent", "proper" and "improper", but form a totally new development without roots in the past. Musallam's book is indelible proof

that Muslim society ... was a whole lot more understanding and "permissive" – to use a modern term – than the situation of today seems to convey'. G. H. A. Juynboll, 'Review of Basim F. Musallam, *Sex and Society in Islam: Birth Control before the Nineteenth Century*', *International Journal of Middle East Studies*, 18.4 (November 1986), 510–11.

Conclusion

Womb to tomb: The afterlives of early medieval women's remedies

In the summer of 2022, I took my family with me for our first visit to the British Museum. After slowly passing through the crowded halls, we finally stepped into room 41, where the centrepiece is the magnificent Sutton Hoo case, filled with treasures: golden buckles, famous helmets, weapons and drinking horns. But that's not why I was there. I had in mind a much smaller item: the Broadstairs Woman, a tiny, naked figure whose head is a 'corroded lump of iron'.[1] As I walked from case to case, desperately scanning the museum catalogue on my cellphone to locate her in this room full of priceless gold objects, I despaired of finding her. I circled the room, worrying more and seeing less with each passing moment. But then my eyes slid over a set of four slivers of metal, and I *knew*, I just *knew* that I had found her.

While I had read about the dimensions of this figure, I had never thought materially about her. Audrey Meaney writes that she is 25 mm long, which is about the length of an ordinary sewing needle, but Meaney's description of her as hanging from a 'girdle hanger' gave me the impression that she was longer, bigger, more substantial, serving as a kind of key chain for a woman of power and authority perhaps. Instead, she is tiny, a private object fitting easily inside a closed fist. I excitedly called my family over, and my youngest daughter asked me to read the description. I read:

> 2. Pagan Imagery: Animals were significant to pagan Anglo-Saxon beliefs. Boars and birds-of-prey often decorated war gear like this helmet fitting and shield ornament. Women's jewellery also featured animals, like the horse-shaped brooch and gold pendant with birds' heads. Naturalistic images of humans were rarer. The four figurines may have been fertility charms, or protective amulets.[2]

She looked at me, confused, and asked were there any birds on the figure. I laughed and explained that no, all that description about animal imagery wasn't about these little figures. And then I stopped laughing as I realised that three of the five sentences of description were not at all about the qualities of this figure, and they described not what she was, but rather what she was not. There was no description of the fact that she was found in a woman's grave in Kent, or that she would have been a worn object because she was found 'suspended from a belt by an iron girdle-hanger, with iron tweezers and a key'.[3] In a room full of men's objects, this woman's object didn't receive even the slightest mention of her unique ownership and identity; she was grouped with other figures both male and female, and received not even a sentence to herself.

The Broadstairs Woman was my first stop on the journey of this book project many years ago. I sat at a table in the Institute for Research in the Humanities at the University of Wisconsin in Madison and looked for the first time at Audrey Meaney's book *Anglo-Saxon Amulets and Curing Stones*. When I turned to page 231, there she was, sketched at two-to-three times her actual size. I read her description greedily. Near the end, Meaney writes:

> She is very unobtrusive in her sexuality, but no-one who handled and looked hard at her could have been unaware of it; and, since she was worn hung from the girdle with keys, it would be very hard to deny that she had some symbolic or amuletic value for her Anglo-Saxon mistress. What her specific function was, it is more difficult to tell. She cannot come into the category of a gross 'anti-Evil Eye' amulet. Most probably, considering her characteristics and her position, she was worn to increase love; or perhaps fertility – although this would seem more likely if the secondary sexual characteristics (the breasts) were emphasized.[4]

I stared at the page in shock. How had I never heard of this figurine? Why was she not more prominently displayed, why not discussed in the texts that explore the lives of medieval women? How had I missed this, on display in the British Museum? How had *we all* overlooked this remarkable object, even though Meaney showed her to us? The Broadstairs Woman, like the bodies of medieval women, is enmeshed in the effacement of early medieval women. The texts exclude, and so readers and scholars exclude, assuming an absence where very often there is one, but also where sometimes there is not.

Certainly the tiny figurine of the Broadstairs Woman and her companion, the Higham Amulet, a 'Copper-alloy three-dimensional amuletic figure in the form of a naked female figure',[5] do not have the show-stopping quality of the Alfred Jewel or the Sutton Hoo Helmet, but is their absence from the larger cultural conversation and imagination because they feature women, rather than kings or warriors? Despite the common belief in early medieval women's absence in representation, here are two amulets featuring naked women, likely connected to fertility and fecundity. These figurines are not so sexualised as the traditional Sheela-na-gig, a fertility amulet with origins in Irish culture. But in light of a literary culture in early medieval England that is far more prudish, that these female figurines exist at all is shocking, made all the more incredible by the fact that they are explicitly naked below the waist, with the vulva of the Broadstairs Woman obviously marked. Although fertility amulets exist widely in female graves of the time, usually in the form of natural items like cowrie shells rather than figural images, these two small figures offer us something that is both ordinary and extraordinary: the tangible bodies of women, worn and owned by women.[6]

Women's absences across Old English culture are repeatedly noted in the scholarly conversation, from the literary tradition, where only one woman speaks in all 3,000 lines of *Beowulf*, to the historical record, wherein both biblical and royal genealogies list only the names of fathers. As Mary Dockray-Miller states,

> In Anglo-Saxon culture at large, both during and after Bede, patrilineage was the focus of most extant genealogy; such a patrilineal focus was also coupled with a usual exclusion of women's roles and names at all, erasing and eliding the biologically crucial maternal body from both the family tree and the historical focus.[7]

Thus, mothers were written out of questions of lineage and out of the literature that perpetuates and reflects this patriarchal culture. What matters, these lineages proclaim, is the father who propagated the offspring, not the body and person who carried and nurtured that life, or who provided it with half of its genetics and familial connections.[8] Alex Traves confirms this bias, but argues for a different pattern in Asser's *Life of King Alfred*, where women are featured far more prominently.[9] Just as with the presence of the Broadstairs Woman, we need not accept the patterns of absence of women in the Old English tradition as a fundamental and undeniable truth. Women existed in early medieval culture, and they exist in the material and literary cultures that survive. Our contemporary practices of belief (and disbelief) take part in the occluding of the bodies and lives of women. As this book has worked to demonstrate, remedies for women exist and speak to the lives and experiences of women, not because of their absence, but because of their presence.

Who's the *mann:* The universal male body and women's medicine

Old English remedies commonly begin with variations of the phrase 'Wiþ þon þe mon …' ('If a man …'), followed by a wide range of problems that might befall this poor person, from bacterial infections to sore eyes to open wounds. Although Bosworth-Toller defines *mann* as 'a human being of either sex', it defines *mannlice* as 'manfully, in a manner becoming to a man, nobly'.[10] Therefore, while anyone might be a *mann*, in truth, that generic noun is crowded out by its overburdened adjective. In Old English, to be *mannlice* is not to be human, but to be masculine. A *mann* is an ideal subject, a person worthy of address, and a body that can be treated for its maladies. It is a recuperable body, and one that can carry forward the markers of desirable behaviour and identity. It is the most human of the human forms, an ideal to be sought after, and one from which to be departed has crucial consequences in terms of health both spiritual and medical.

But how should we read the word *mann/mon* in the remedies? Any person might experience the majority of maladies that appear in the leechbooks, and so it seems reasonable to think of the term *mann* in a general sense. And yet the word fundamentally implies the male, even in its neutral form, which, as Christine Rauer notes, 'is more closely associated with male than with female gender'.[11] Kathryn Maude similarly argues, in a discussion of homilies, that '*Mann* is an exclusionary term, and cannot always be assumed to include the listening women in Ælfric's audience.'[12] So the question is, when the medical texts offer remedies for *mann*, are women part of the intended audience?

One remedy suggests a possible answer: in remedy thirty-seven of *Bald*, the author discusses *at length* the many methods to address urine retention. The passage offers fourteen potential methods, seven times using the word *mon* in order to describe the sufferer, while also employing variations of phrasing like 'Eft' ('Again') to indicate a new method, or occasionally 'Wiþ þon ilcan eft' ('For the same again').[13] The passage includes four occurrences of *he*, the masculine singular pronoun, to reference this same sufferer. None of this is particularly remarkable or unusual in the structure of remedies. What *is* remarkable, however, is the thirteenth method, which specifies 'Gif wif ne mæge gemigan nim tuncerran sæd seoð on wætre sele drincan' ('If a woman cannot urinate, take seed of garden cress, boil it in water and give it to drink').[14] This method is immediately followed by the final entry for the section, which returns the formulation to *mann*: 'Gif mon ne mæge gemigan …' ('If a man cannot urinate …').[15] It seems that perhaps there is something specific to a woman's iteration of this malady that requires a different treatment, and that cannot be applied to a man. If that is so, then we might similarly posit that remedies for men were meant to treat men. Women might use these remedies, but the remedies were not established with them in mind.

The *LBIII* also includes a remedy that distinguishes between male and female recipients, and while it relies on a generic form of *mann*, it does so with the specific aim to distinguish between treatments for men and women. The remedy for 'elf hiccups' begins 'Gif him biþ ælfsogoþa …' ['If an elf hiccup is for him …'], using the masculine singular pronoun both in this moment and later in the passage in its nominative form.[16] Following the initial descriptor of the disease, the remedy calls on the physician to observe the person seeking help, specifically identifying their sex and differentiating symptoms for men and women:

> Gif þu þone *mon* lacnian wille þænc *his* gebæra 7 wite hwilces hades *he* sie. Gif hit biþ *wæpned man* 7 locað up þonne þu *hine* ærest sceawast 7 se anwlita biþ geolwe blac. Þone *mon* þu meaht gelacnian æltæwlice gif *he* ne biþ þær on to lange. Gif hit biþ *wif* 7 locað niþer þonne þu *hit* ærest sceawast. 7 *hire* anwlita biþ reade wan þæt þu miht eac gelacnian.

[If you wish to cure the *man*, think about *his* bearing and see of what kind of man *he* might be. If it is a *weaponed-man* and looks up when you first see *him* and the face is yellow black, you can cure the *man* completely if *he* is not ill for too long. If it is a *woman* and looks down when you first see *it*, and *her* face is dark red, you can also cure that.][17]

I have emphasised the paired gendered nouns and pronouns in this passage in order to show the strangeness of the grammatical constructions around sex, but also to indicate how these terms ultimately indicate male referents. The first occurrences of *hine* (him) and *mon* (person/man) might function as generics, noting that the physician must determine which *hades* (rank/type/condition) the *mon* is – in other words, what *kind* of man is the man. The options are either a man-man, using the term *wæpned* to highlight the masculinity of the man, or a *wif* (woman).[18] This translation might seem hyperbolic – after all, we are meant to understand the word *mann* as a general term for person, but I would suggest that even in its most innocuous state, the word for person indicates the male body as the default body, and this remedy offers no exception.

Even as the remedy indicates a distinction between the way it affects the male body and the female one, it highlights the male as its baseline by listing that body first, and then setting the female body as a contrast. Furthermore, the continued use of the masculine pronoun to refer both to the generic body of the *mann* and to the male body of the *wæpned man* ('weaponed man') suggests that there is virtually no difference between them. Notably, in this example, the feminine pronoun occurs only once, and an occurrence of the neuter pronoun *hit* is used to describe the woman, when in the parallel passage for the man, the masculine pronoun *hine* is used. Therefore, it is the woman who becomes the neuter example, while the male patient retains his masculine status even before his *hades* ('kind') is determined.

Bald, too, calls for the physician to consider the nature of the individual body when suggesting treatment. In Section 35, the author offers treatment for a 'asweartedum 7 adeadedum lice' ('darkened and decaying body').[19] While the majority of remedies are brief, this remedy is extensive, almost three folio pages long (from fols 31a to 32a), and, about halfway through, offers advice that, while specific to this treatment, also seems relevant as advice to the physician in other circumstances: 'Do þu þa læcedomas swilce þu þa lichoman gesie. For þon ðe micel gedal gif on wæpnedes 7 wifes 7 cildes lichoman' ('You should do the leechdom appropriate to the body you observe, because of the great distinction between the bodies of weaponed ones and women and children').[20] The author continues, suggesting that the physician should consider the physical differences between the old and the young; the labourer and the idle person; the people who are black, white and red, as well. The remedy here, and perhaps all remedies, are meant for all bodies, with adjustments to their specific physical qualities. However, the remedy relies on a general form, a default body, and that body is neither a female body, nor a childlike one. The default body in this remedy, and perhaps in any remedy for a *mann*, is an adult male body: a body that is understood as average; a body that is understood as *not female*.

The fundamental misogyny of the medieval medical system, a system that treats the male body as the ideal form, offers few remedies specific to women. This is particularly ironic given the danger women experienced as a result of reproductive problems. In fact, a simple look at proportions gives us statistics that demonstrate exactly this. In a count of those remedies included in the three volumes of *Leechdoms, Wortcunning, and Starcraft of Early England*, Cockayne includes approximately 1,516 distinct remedies. He occasionally omits remedies that offend his Victorian sensibilities, and so we must assume additional unique remedies. In a search of the *DOE Web Corpus*, the word *wif* occurs 111 times across all of the possible remedies, but these occurrences do not reflect the number of remedies specific to women, as often *wif* occurs multiple times in a single remedy, and sometimes *wif* is used to modify the word milk, as breastmilk was an occasional ingredient in general remedies. In a non-exhaustive search of the same remedies, without accounting for variations in the vowel or multiple occurrences in a single remedy, the word *mon* occurs 287 times *at least*. *Wæpned* occurs only nine times in these same texts. If we were to assumed that the *only* remedies that were specifically for men were those that use the phrase *wæpned man*, then it would be true that there are more remedies for women than for men. Rather, I suggest that any remedy for *mann/mon* is a remedy directed to the generic male body, with the use of *wæpned* likely serving to distinguish, as above, between 'kinds' of men, rather than to be the primary marker of the male body. Indeed, if we return to the statistics, assuming there are upwards of 1,500 remedies total, only approximately fifty of these remedies are specific to women's concerns, and so less than 3 per cent of the total remedies treat women explicitly.[21]

Women almost assuredly did benefit from the general set of remedies, but they were not identified as or understood to be the ideal target. And this omission matters, because we know now that women experience illness and disease differently than men do. Contemporary medical research still treats the male body as the default body, which endangers the lives of women now, as it likely did then. Caroline Criado Perez argues vehemently for the need to treat and research women's bodies as different from men's, saying:

> For millennia, medicine has functioned on the assumption that male bodies can represent humanity as a whole. As a result, we have a huge historical data gap when it comes to female bodies, and this is a data gap that is continuing to grow as researchers carry on ignoring the pressing ethical need to include female cells, animals and humans, in their research. That this is still going on in the twenty-first century is a scandal. It should be the subject of newspaper headlines worldwide. Women are dying, and the medical world is complicit. It needs to wake up.[22]

Treatments aimed at the generalised body were and are not treatments that consider women's specific symptoms. But every single remedy that does not specify that it is for women *is* for men.

Menopause in the early medieval medical tradition

So often, the women's remedies that do exist are remedies that serve the community and facilitate social function; in other words, they are remedies that serve both men and women in the ways that they treat women's bodies. Remedies for menstruation, for fertility, for childbirth, for miscarriage and for abortion are remedies that address women's needs but also family needs. Each of these categories serves reproductive purposes, whether they work to bring on irregular menstrual cycles so that a woman can conceive, or clear away a miscarriage, stillbirth or unwanted pregnancy. What no remedy does, explicitly, is to treat postfertile women's bodies.

Conceptually, menopause and language for it are absent in early medieval remedies, but this omission does not suggest that the condition itself did not exist or impact women. The word 'menopause' was only coined in 1821 by a French physician, Charles-Pierre-Louis de Gardanne, although its symptoms began to appear in written medical discussions around 1700.[23] It is certain that early medieval women experienced the cessation of menses, likely in their forties and fifties, but we don't know what that experience looked like or meant for them.[24] Physicians and researchers Ricki Pollicove, Frederick Naftolin and James A. Simon offer a list of common menopausal symptoms, including cardiovascular disease, hypertension, arteriosclerosis, osteoporosis, scarring and genital atrophy, hot flashes, night sweats, sleep disorders, memory deficiency, impaired cognition, and cancer.[25] While not all women experience all of these symptoms, they are common enough to be consistently listed and understood as standard markers of menopause. While these symptoms likely would have impacted early medieval women's health, no remedies for women seem to address any of these concerns explicitly.

Perhaps this absence of remedies has to do with early medieval women's life spans – in other words, perhaps women did not live long enough to experience menopause in meaningful ways. Nick Stoodley locates the life expectancy of early medieval English women at thirty,[26] but Duncan Sayer and Sam D. Dickinson note that this number is likely skewed by the high rate of maternal mortality, which disproportionately affects women in their twenties and thirties; importantly, they explain that Stoodley's

> statistics are derived from skeletal data so suffer from a tendency to underrepresent older individuals and ignore skeletons which could not be sexed ... However, the results are conspicuous, placing over 38 per cent of Anglo-Saxon female mortality into a single decade of life, a trend unlikely to be the product solely of sampling error. A pattern this striking ... is likely to have maternal mortality as its dynamic factor.[27]

What we have, then, are data demonstrating that women were very likely to die as a result of complications from childbirth, and scholarship looks to these significant trends. That does not mean, however, that women did not survive past age thirty; in fact, Stoodley's data, impacted as it is by uncertainty regarding some remains, still shows that more than thirty women out of '374 female skeletons from 46 cemeteries' lived to be between forty and fifty or older.[28] Indeed, Sayer suggests 'Although there is no evidence to suggest that the maximum extent of life in the past was any shorter than it is today, the chance of reaching that extent was reduced significantly.'[29] While 10 per cent of the population is not an enormous amount, we must assume that a reasonable proportion of women reached an age where they might experience the symptoms of menopause.

Perhaps no early medieval remedies for menopause exist because early medieval people did not experience significant symptoms on account of a physically demanding lifestyle. Pollycove, Naftolin and Simon suggest that:

> Because hunter-gatherers are extremely vigorous and active even through the late menopause years, they are likely to have been among the least bothered by menopausal symptoms, as evidenced by data on sleep disorders in women from less developed nations as compared with sedentary women in post-industrial countries.[30]

Early medieval levels of physical activity and diet might differ in significant ways from contemporary capitalist social systems, but they likely also differed significantly from hunter-gatherer societies. We cannot assume that because early medieval women did not work at desks and drive cars they might not have been impacted by potentially debilitating symptoms of menopause. Just as telling contemporary people to change their diets and exercise patterns does not fundamentally resolve the effects of menopause, we cannot assume that a more active lifestyle and lower caloric diet of women in the Middle Ages would have exempted them from the experience of physical exhaustion, declining mental acuity, and hot flashes and night sweats brought on by radically shifting hormones.

Perhaps, more than anything else, early medieval women might have had very different expectations for ageing. Perhaps the lack of remedies results not from shame and disregard – problems that have impacted research on menopause in contemporary culture for far too long – but rather from people's acceptance that to be of a certain age is necessarily accompanied by these kinds of physical decline. Perhaps people simply expected and accepted these physiological experiences without turning to a medical tradition to help them manage their physical symptoms.

While having little expectation that the medical tradition would address unpleasant symptoms of ageing is entirely possible, a group of remedies suggests that this acceptance of the limitation of age might not be the same for women and men: remedies for what we might understand today as erectile dysfunction. The Old English medical tradition includes more remedies for erectile dysfunction than for childbirth. The *Medicina de Quadrupedibus* (*OEM*) includes six remedies for erectile dysfunction (and, to be fair, one remedy for women's pleasure). As I noted in the introduction to this book, contemporary research for erectile dysfunction receives five times more funding than research into endometriosis; this same prioritisation of extended male sex identity and function is present in the Old English tradition.[31] The Old English remedies for men suggest such ingredients as boar and goat gall, bull testicles, and deer faeces and testicles, and most seek to imbue the man with the vigour of the animal whose parts he uses as treatment. Here, the goal seems to be to transfer the lust of the boar into the body of the man, via the application of its smeared effluvia: 'Were wylla to gefremmanne: nime bares geallan ond smyre mid þone teors ond þa hærþan. Þonne hafað he mycelne lust' ('For a man's desire to perform: take boar's gall and smear the penis and testicles. Then he will have great lust').[32] The goal of the remedy is to induce lust in the seeker, and while we cannot prove this remedy only works to treat older men who have lost their virility due to ageing, contemporary statistics suggest 'that ED is increasingly prevalent with age: approximately 40% of men are affected at age 40 and nearly 70% of men are affected at age 70'.[33] Treatments for virility in men likely target the effect of ageing on men's ability to perform sexually, even after their prime – whereas women in menopause might well have seen the experience to be part of their progression through ageing and on the decline toward death in a way that would not have been mitigated or improved by treatment. The medieval medical tradition, much like the contemporary one, offers more care and concern for ageing male bodies than female ones.

Lament as we might the paucity of treatments for women's maladies in the medical tradition, the lack of care for ageing women is even more glaring. Of the tiny number of remedies for women, two are so broad that they do not fit neatly into any identifiable category, like menstrual woes or fertility issues. We might be tempted to see them as remedies for the symptoms of menopause, but their vagueness makes this identification almost impossible. The two Old English remedies from the *OEM* use a similar generic phrase to offer palliative care for women: *wið wifa earfoðnyssum* ('for women's afflictions'). The first of these occurrences includes a garbled Latin phrase that Conan Doyle and Christine Voth identify as a reference to '*hysterica pnix* or "hysterical strangulation", a condition in which the womb is believed to have moved up into the chest seeking out blood or moisture'.[34] The remedy offers little information about the condition itself:

> Wif wifa earfoðnyssum, þas uncyste Grecas hatað *hystem cepnizam*: heortes hornes þæs smælestan dustes bruce; þry dagas on wines drince. Gif he feforig sy, drince þonne on wearmum wætere. Þæt bið god læcecræft
>
> [For women's afflictions, the disorder the Greeks call *hystem cepnizam*: use the most finely ground powder of deer horn; drink it in wine for three days. If this person is feverish, drink in warm water. That is a good remedy.][35]

The ingredient here offers no help in determining the symptoms the remedy purports to treat: deer antler is used to 'ælcne wætan adrigenne' ('dry up each wetness'),[36] but is also for headache, loose teeth, excessive menstruation, killing worms and snakes, spleen pain, and impetigo. The only symptom the remedy includes is fever, and even that is an ancillary possibility rather than an identifying factor. Conan Doyle connects this remedy with a gloss that identifies the malady as a blocking of the womb, but that descriptor is of little help, given the general precept of 'drying up'.

The second of the two remedies is similarly confounding, although a secondary ingredient may have some connections with homoeopathic treatments for menopause. This remedy calls for an ointment to be applied on or perhaps even inside a woman's body:

> Wið wifa earfoðnyssum þe on heora inwerdlicum stowum earfeþu þrowiað: foxes leoþu ond his smeoru, mid ealdon ele ond mid tyrwan; wyrc him to sealfe; do on wifa stowe. Hraþe hit þa earfeþu gehæleþ.

[For women's affliction, who experience pain in their inward places: mix fox's limbs and fat with old oil and tar; work them into a salve and apply on the woman's place. It will heal the pain almost immediately.][37]

Tar might seem at first to be an off-putting ingredient, but pine tar (unlike coal tar) is an ingredient that 'has been shown to be anti-pruritic, anti-inflammatory, antibacterial and antifungal', and has 'been used in medicine for more than 2,000 years to treat a range of skin conditions because of its soothing and antiseptic properties'.[38] Thus, a remedy that might initially appear merely bizarre might very well have worked to soothe and heal inflamed body parts. Indeed, pine tar serves as a common ingredient in contemporary homoeopathic treatments for menopause, and particularly rosacea, which is sometimes called menopausal acne and may be triggered by hot flashes and hormone fluctuations.[39] But this remedy does not suggest the treatment is exactly topical, or for one's complexion: rather, it seems to be genital, and so although the ingredients are consistent with menopause symptoms, the indications for use here – likely either external to or perhaps even inside the vagina – suggest a different set of concerns. Perhaps it works as a treatment for vaginal dryness; perhaps 'wifa stowe' ('woman's place') has no particularly gynaecological register – but this seems unlikely. Therefore, unlike the childbirth remedies, we find no clear answer as to whether the category of 'women's afflictions' might suggest common symptoms of menopause.

In some ways, these remedies fall into the convenient and familiar category of 'lady troubles', a euphemistic way of dismissing or generalising women's real maladies. But perhaps this language merely *appears* euphemistic. As Roberta Frank has argued in her discussion of the Old English language for sex, the *DOE* must work to achieve 'the almost impossible task of balancing the Anglo-Saxon writer's delicate sense of propriety and register with the modern reader's conviction that pussyfooted euphemisms are themselves obscene'.[40] What we encounter here is nothing that seems obscene, but rather is familiarly vague, and we are all too content to accept that nebulousness as the same kind of ambiguity we use in contemporary language. But perhaps the language on the page is less about what Frank thinks of as 'propriety' and more what she means by 'register'. We are simply unable to interpret the register; we do not have adequate information. Perhaps these remedies might have spoken to a known category of women's suffering; we cannot know if they were intended to treat the symptoms of menopause.

Conclusions: The matter of language and why language matters

The logic of this book has been to work through and think about the language of women's medicine in Old English, starting with menstruation, moving through remedies for fertility, pregnancy, childbirth, miscarriage, cleansing, purging and abortion. While certain categories here might share properties with menopause, there seems to be no specific language that invokes this age or experience for early medieval English woman. The medicine that appears in the textual tradition seems not to consider this phase of life as one worthy of attention, or even to understand it as a quasi-universal set of symptoms that could be anticipated or treated.

The 'hysteric philology' I established in the introduction of this book both does and does not speak to this problem of menopause. Hysteric philology is a practice by which close attention to language breaks apart the tidy but inaccurate veneer of polite inattention to the specific elements of women's medicine. This approach values the lives and bodies of ordinary, not just extraordinary, women, finding those women in the remedies as they call out for medical attention, share their symptoms and request help. The voices of the wise, experienced, sweating survivors – the women who did not die in childbirth – do not find purchase in the medical tradition. They slide away, and perhaps we can find echoes of them here and there: in the *Lacnunga* remedies for 'cardiacus, hatte seo adl ðe man swiðe swæteð' ('cardiacus, what the illness is called when a man sweats heavily'),[41] or 'Slæp-drænc' ('sleep-drink'), a concoction of radish, hemlock, wormwood and henbane that might well have helped someone sleep a little *too* well.[42] We could search the remedies to see what kinds of treatments might have helped individual complaints commonly associated with menopause, but in truth, we won't find women there, not unless those complaints are specifically gynaecological, and most likely menstrual.

Chapter 1 discusses remedies for menstruation, both in the desire to bring on missing or delayed menses, and in the need to end excessive cycles. Both of these conditions might have affected menopausal women. Irregularity in menstrual cycles is a common complaint, and particularly challenging for perimenopausal people, who, in addition to missing cycles, sometimes experience prolonged or excessive bleeding. The remedies for stopping excessive flow might well speak to these symptoms, including the remedies from London, British Library, MS Royal 2.A.xx that call out in Latin, either implicitly or explicitly, for Veronica, wherein her weeping body facilitates the cessation of her bleeding: 'Fletu riganti supplicis, / arent fluenta sanguinis' ('By the flowing tears of the suppliant / the floods of blood dry up'), and perhaps, even more vigorously, 'Beronice, libera me sanguinibus, Deus, Deus salutis meae' ('Veronica, free me from hemorrhages. God, God of my salvation').[43] These menstrual remedies might well have given comfort to menopausal women, as well as to women suffering from menorrhagia.

Chapter 2, although about issues of fertility and pregnancy, is also very much about the ways in which expert physicians, often men, seek to read and thus circumscribe the bodies of women. Questions of fertility and pregnancy often eddy around the issue of time, wherein the right thing must happen at the right time in order for conception to occur, or to yield the desired kind of conception. Similarly, remedies and prognostics for pregnancy seek to demystify the pregnant body, and to understand, in a sense *before* the appointed time, the nature of the foetus carried inside. The authors of such texts often figure women as ignorant of the processes inside their own bodies, whose behaviours and choices can either manifest truths about the foetus or write characteristics on the malleable body inside via their own personal appetites. In a sense, these unreadable bodies speak to the unreadable bodies of menopausal and perimenopausal people, whose relation to time and fertility is similarly vexed and uncertain. As with both conception and pregnancy, menopause offers a kind of threshold – a boundary that separates the fertile body from the body that no longer can, or perhaps even must, bear children. The perimenopausal body is one that can still conceive, but one whose workings are obscure, even to the person who inhabits it, for at least a time. Is the cessation of a menstrual cycle a sign of conception, or of the lack of even the possibility of conception? Only time can reveal this answer.

Chapter 3 focuses closely on issues of language around childbirth, working to disentangle terms that have too often been understood to signify a single experience, and which generalise the totality of conception through childbirth as a single and unified event. This chapter itself was conceived from the paucity of remedies for childbirth. The lack of such remedies puzzled me, particularly given the urgent danger presented to medieval women, as demonstrated by the mortuary evidence. How could a culture that lost so many women to this event not even attempt medically to treat their bodies *in extremis*, I wondered. I found that language around childbirth was more complex and also more specific than many translations and dictionaries had revealed. I wonder if this same operation might be true, too, for menopausal bodies. Certainly a unified term for this experience is too much to expect, particularly at a time when only a small proportion of the population would have lived to experience menopause.

When I first began this project, I suspected that the category of purging and cleansing might apply to ageing women's bodies, but in the process of composing Chapter 4, I determined that these procedures are more often connected with miscarriage, stillbirth and abortion. This is not to say that menopausal women never sought cleansing or purging in response to changes in menstruation, but none of the remedies in this category registers this set of concerns directly. Might women have used such remedies to seek physiological and gynaecological balance? Certainly. But, as Chapter 4 argues, the womb is being cleansed of something quite specific, and that matter is frequently foetal tissue. If people were using these remedies later in life to address their particular symptoms, they would have been applying the general principle of the remedy as opposed to something directly indicated by the remedy itself.

This final chapter, and the book as a whole, offer a glimpse into the kinds of lives and choices ordinary medieval women might have had relative to their medical status and gynaecological conditions. Reducing people to their genitals is generally a losing proposition, yet in many ways the genitals are the only way in which women appear differentiated in medical texts. The default body, the male body, does not menstruate, conceive or give birth, and so remedies for men cannot speak to these specific concerns of women. Not all women could or did (or wanted to) reproduce, and so in invoking reproductive or conceiving bodies in my title, I do not invoke the necessity of reproduction. If anything, this text has shown that women might well have wanted to and attempted to exert control over their reproductive destiny. These same freedoms, granted by amorphous language and the perceived timing of conception and ensoulment, are not granted to many people in contemporary culture given contemporary laws around abortion, privacy and medical rights.

The popular contemporary perception of the Middle Ages is as a time of violence, absolute religious obedience and laughable medical treatment, with no rights or autonomy for women. The notion that we, in contemporary culture, are nothing like our medieval counterparts is an exaggeration of both their primitive beliefs and practices, and our allegedly evolved ones. The consequences of medical beliefs and ideologies are all too often visited upon the bodies of people at the mercy of their reproductive status. Medieval graveyards are populated by far too many women who died as a result of pregnancy, childbirth or its complications. Let us strive to avoid the same fate for contemporary bodies.

Notes

1 Audrey Meaney, *Anglo-Saxon Amulets and Curing Stones* (Oxford: British Archaeological Reports, 1981), p. 231.
2 British Museum placard, found in room 41. She is difficult to find via the museum's website, which directs one to the Odin figurine and the Higham amulet, which is in better condition. The Higham Amulet's location is identified as museum number 2001, 0711.1, on display (G41/dc6/SB).
3 Meaney, *Anglo-Saxon Amulets*, p. 231.
4 Ibid., p. 238.
5 The objects may be seen respectively at www.britishmuseum.org/collection/object/H_2001-0711-1 and www.britishmuseum.org/collection/object/H_1988-0412-1 (both accessed 27 October 2021).
6 Women's graves frequently include amuletic objects according to Meaney, *Anglo-Saxon Amulets*, pp. 232–8. These amuletic objects often invoke fertility-related protections, as Helen Geake notes in her discussion of cowrie shells, which 'are used all over the world as

amulets, because of their resemblance to different things. The usual explanation is that the underside looks like a human vulva, and therefore the shell must have been an aid to fertility. In Anglo-Saxon graves, cowrie shells are found almost exclusively with women of child-bearing age and children. ' Helen Geake, 'The Use of Grave-Goods in Conversion Period England c. 600–c.850 A.D.', 2 vols, PhD thesis (University of York, 1995), p. 142.

7 Mary Dockray-Miller, *Motherhood and Mothering in Anglo-Saxon England* (London: Palgrave Macmillan, 2000), p. xiii.

8 'Despite the large body of extant royal genealogies from this period, overwhelmingly they document men, mostly kings, and trace descent patrilineally, ignoring maternal ancestors and the genealogies of royal women.' Alex Traves, 'Genealogy and Royal Women in Asser' s Life of King Alfred: Politics, Prestige, and Maternal Kinship in Early Medieval England', *Early Medieval Europe*, 30.1 (2022), 101–24 (p. 104).

9 Ibid., pp. 123–4.

10 Joseph Bosworth, 'mann' and 'mann-líce', in *An Anglo-Saxon Dictionary Online*, ed. Thomas Northcote Toller, Christ Sean and Ondřej Tichy (Prague: Faculty of Arts, Charles University, 2014), https://bosworthtoller.com/22366 (accessed 23 December 2023).

11 Christine Rauer, '*Mann* and Gender in Old English Prose', *Neophilologus*, 131 (2017), 139–58 (p. 140). Kathryn Maude, in a discussion of men's addresses to women in religious letters and sermons, discusses the limits of the words *mann* and *breðren*, which can both function as generic terms, to refer to groups that include both men and women, suggesting that while they *can* work as generic terms, in many instances they do not. *Addressing Women in Early Medieval Religious Texts* (Woodbridge: Boydell and Brewer, 2021), pp. 22–9.

12 Maude, *Addressing Women*, p. 24.

13 Thomas Oswald Cockayne, *Leechdoms, wortcunning, and starcraft of early England. Being a collection of documents, for the most part never before printed, illustrating the history of science in this country before the Norman Conquest*, 3 vols (London: Longman, Green, Longman, Roberts and Green, 1864–66), Vol. II, p. 88.

14 Ibid., Vol. II, p. 90. He even adds an extra feminine pronoun in his translation, saying 'give it *to her* to drink' (p. 91; emphasis mine).

15 Ibid., Vol. II, p. 90. Interestingly, in his own translation of this passage, Cockayne shifts to the gender-neutral 'one', despite using 'man' as the translation term for the previous part of entry 37 consistently.

16 The grammatical formulation here is strange, even in terms of the regular diagnostic language. The pronoun functions as a masculine

singular, the verb as a third-person-singular indicative, and the noun as a weak masculine singular. Bosworth-Toller offers both 'hiccup' and 'heartburn' as possible descriptions of this singular malady. Many thanks to Erin Sweany for helping me untangle this vexed passage.

17 Cockayne, *Leechdoms*, Vol. II, p. 348, Chapter lxii.
18 I have discussed the notion of a 'weaponed man' in my first book, *Monsters, Gender, and Sexuality in Medieval English Literature* (Woodbridge: Boydell and Brewer, 2010), noting the ways in which adding the first term highlights the masculinity of the second. There, I draw on the term *wæpenwifestre* ('weaponed woman'), which is glossed as 'hermaphrodite', suggesting that a woman who is weaponed is one who has taken on phallic properties of masculinity.
19 Cockayne, *Leechdoms*, Vol. II, p. 82.
20 Ibid., Vol. II, p. 84.
21 This count does not include the header, which functions like an index of remedies, but just the individual remedies themselves. In some cases, the tables of contents include remedies that do not exist because some folios are missing, as with *Bald*'s table of contents.
22 Caroline Criado Perez, *Invisible Women: Data Bias in a World Designed for Men* (New York: Abrams Press, 2019), pp. 323–4.
23 Susan P. Mattern, 'A Time of Change: A History of Our Understanding of the Menopause. How Has the Way in which We Understand the Menopause Evolved over Time?', *History Matters* (28 June 2021), www.historyextra.com/period/20th-century/a-time-of-change-understanding-menopause (accessed 6 June 2023).
24 In evolutionary terms, researchers continue to debate when menopause as a variably packaged set of physiological experiences began to occur, but they generally agree that 'it is likely to have evolved since the time of the last common ancestor', meaning that menopause is specifically part of the human condition. Ricki Pollycove, Frederick Naftolin and James A. Simon, 'The Evolutionary Origin and Significance of Menopause', *Menopause*, 18.3 (2011): 336–42, DOI: 10.1097/gme.0b013e3181ed957a, p. 338.
25 Ibid.
26 N. Stoodley, 'Multiple Burials, Multiple Meanings? Interpreting the Early Anglo-Saxon Multiple Interment', in S. Lucy and A. Reynolds (eds), *Burial in Early Medieval England and Wales* (Leeds: Society for Medieval Archaeology, 2002), pp. 103–21 (p. 119).
27 Duncan Sayer and Sam D. Dickinson, 'Reconsidering Obstetric Death and Female Fertility in Anglo-Saxon England', *World Archaeology*, 45.2 (2013), 285–97 (p. 293).
28 Ibid.

29 Duncan Sayer, 'Death and the Family: Developing a Generational Chronology', *Journal of Social Archaeology*, 10.1 (2010), 59–91 (p. 65).
30 Pollycove et al., 'Evolutionary Origin', p. 338.
31 Nicola Slawson, '"Women Have Been Woefully Neglected": Does Medical Science Have a Gender Problem?', *Guardian* (18 December 2019), www.theguardian.com/education/2019/dec/18/women-have-been-woefully-neglected-does-medical-science-have-a-gender-problem (accessed 3 November 2021).
32 John P. Niles and Maria D'Aronco (eds and trans), *Anglo-Saxon Medical Texts*, Vol. I, *The Old English Herbal, Lacnunga, and Other Texts*, Dumbarton Oaks Medieval Library (Cambridge: Harvard University Press, 2023), p. 402 (9.8).
33 Milton Lakin and Hadley Wood, 'Erectile Dysfunction', Cleveland Clinic Center for Continuing Education (2018), www.clevelandclinicmeded.com/medicalpubs/diseasemanagement/endocrinology/erectile-dysfunction (accessed 12 June 2023).
34 Christine Voth, 'Women and "Women's Medicine", Early Medieval England: From Text to Practice', in R. Trilling, R. Norris and R. Stephenson (eds), *Feminist Approaches to Anglo-Saxon Studies* (Amsterdam: Amsterdam University Press, 2023), pp. 279–316 (p. 289). Conan Doyle traces the roots of this phrase, ultimately suggesting 'This Greek term, ὑστερικὴ πνίξ meaning "suffocation of the womb" is one of the most garbled Greek terms in the Old English Herbal, the word division having been misconstrued by a scribe at some point in the transmission history, and later scribes further attempting to create two new words in the accusative, resulting in the gibberish hystem cepnizam in Sextus Placitus α, i.7, transcribed letter for letter as such by the Anglo-Saxon scribe of the Medicina de quadrupedibus 3.7. The sense is not lost completely, in no small part due to the presence of the Latin gloss "Mulier si a uulua offocatur" (if a woman be blocked in the womb) translated into Old English as "Wið wifa earfodnyssum" (for the tribulations of women).' Conan Doyle, 'Anglo-Saxon Medicine and Disease: A Semantic Approach', 2 vols, PhD thesis (University of Cambridge, 2011), p. 214.
35 Niles and D'Aronco, *Anglo-Saxon Medical Texts*, Vol. I, p. 376 (3.7).
36 Ibid., p. 376 (3.1).
37 Ibid., p. 380 (4.1).
38 Tanya M. Barnes and Kerryn A. Greive, 'Topical Pine Tar: History, Properties and Use as a Treatment for Common Skin Conditions', *The Australian Journal of Dermatology*, 58.2 (2017), 80–5, DOI: 10.1111/ajd.12427.

39 A simple internet search for pine tar and menopause reveals a range of products targeting menopause, including soaps, serums and salves. See Ananya Mandal, 'Rosacea and Menopause', *NewsMedical Life Sciences* (20 January 2023), www.news-medical.net/health/Rosacea-and-Menopause.aspx (accessed 13 June 2023).

40 Roberta Frank, 'Sex in the Dictionary of Old English', in Mark Amodio and Katherine O'Brien O'Keeffe (eds), *Unlocking the Wordhord: Anglo-Saxon Studies in Memory of Edward B. Irving, Jr.* (Toronto: University of Toronto Press, 2003), pp. 302–12 (p. 304).

41 Niles and D'Aronco, *Anglo-Saxon Medical Texts*, Vol. I, p. 428 (*Lacnunga* 21).

42 Ibid., p. 448 (*Lacnunga* 62).

43 Ibid., pp. 632–3, 636–7, translations theirs.

Bibliography

Abernathy, Susan, 'Edith of Wessex, Queen of England'. www.medievalists.net/2013/02/edith-of-wessex-queen-of-england/ (accessed 27 June 2022).

Adams, Janey, 'Old Wives' Tales, Debunked', NPR. www.npr.org/sections/babyproject/2011/08/02/138549731/old-wives-tales-debunked (accessed 3 March 2020).

Ælfric, *Ælfric's Lives of Saints*, ed. W. W. Skeat, trans. Miss Gunning and Miss Wilkinson, 2 vols, Early English Text Society, o.s. 114 (London: Kegan, Paul, Trench, Trübner, 1900).

Allam, Nida, 'Ectopic Pregnancies Are Medical Emergencies – Not Political Footballs', *Teen Vogue* (1 April 2022). www.teenvogue.com/story/ectopic-pregnancy-abortion (accessed 24 June 2022).

Allegro, John Marco, *The Sacred Mushroom and the Cross* (London: Hodder and Stoughton, 1970).

Almendrala, Anna, 'Why Do Conservatives Still Think Contraception Is Abortion?', *Huffpost Health* (7 September 2018). www.huffpost.com/entry/conservatives-contraception-abortion_n_5b92fd41e4b0cf7b003fc28a (accessed 3 March 2020).

American Pregnancy Association, 'D&C Procedure after a Miscarriage'. https://americanpregnancy.org/pregnancy-complications/d-and-c-procedure-after-miscarriage/#:~:text=A%20D%26C%2C%20also%20known%20as,the%20contents%20of%20the%20uterus (accessed 3 June 2020).

Babbar, Karan, Jennifer Martin, Josephine Ruiz, Ateeb Ahmad Parray and Marni Sommer, 'Menstrual Health Is a Public Health and Human Rights Issue', *The Lancet: Public Health* (27 October 2021). DOI: 10.1016/S2468-2667(21)00212-7 (accessed 17 July 2023).

Barnes, Tanya M. and Kerryn A. Greive, 'Topical Pine Tar: History, Properties and Use as a Treatment for Common Skin Conditions', *The Australian Journal of Dermatology*, 58.2 (2017), 80–85. DOI: 10.1111/ajd.12427.

Barrow, Bill, 'Alabama Governor Invokes God in Banning Nearly All Abortions', AP News (16 May 2019). https://apnews.com/article/7a47ddc761dc4b72a017b0836da3a87b (accessed 6 July 2023).

Batten, Caroline R., '"Lazarus, Come Forth": Pregnancy and Childbirth in the Life Course of Early Medieval English Women', in Thijs Porck and Harriet Soper (eds), *Early Medieval English Life Courses: Cultural-Historical Perspectives* (Leiden: Brill, 2022), pp. 140–58.

Beck, Julie, 'Women Astronauts: To Menstruate or Not to Menstruate', *The Atlantic* (21 April 2016). www.theatlantic.com/health/archive/2016/04/menstruating-in-space/479229/ (accessed 25 July 2022).

Bede, *The Old English Version of Bede's Ecclesiastical History of the English People*, ed. and trans. Thomas Miller, Early English Text Society (Oxford: Oxford University Press, 1959 (1890)).

Beechy, Tiffany, *The Poetics of Old English* (Farnham: Ashgate, 2011).

Bierbaumer, Peter and Hans Sauer, with Helmut W. Klug and Ulrike Krischke (eds), *Dictionary of Old English Plant Names* (2007–09). http://oldenglish-plantnames.org (accessed 19 July 2023).

Blei, Daniela, 'The History of Talking about Miscarriage', *The Cut* (23 April 2018). www.thecut.com/2018/04/the-history-of-talking-about-miscarriage.html (accessed 2 December 2021).

Boddington, Andy, 'Raunds, Northamptonshire: Analysis of a Country Churchyard', *World Archaeology*, 18.3 (February 1987), 411–25.

Bonser, Wilfrid, *The Medical Background of Anglo-Saxon England* (London: Publications of the Wellcome Historical Library, 1963).

Bosworth, Joseph, *An Anglo-Saxon Dictionary Online*, ed. Thomas Northcote Toller, Christ Sean and Ondřej Tichy (Prague: Faculty of Arts, Charles University, 2014). https://bosworthtoller.com/ (accessed 23 December 2023).

Brackmann, Rebecca, '"It Will Help Him Wonderfully": Placebo and Meaning Responses in Early Medieval English Medicine', *Speculum*, 97.4 (2022), 1012–39.

Brown, G. H., 'Solving the "Solve" Riddle in BL, MS Harley 585', *Viator*, 18 (1989), 45–51.

Brundle, Lisa, 'The Body on Display: Exploring the Role and Use of Figurines in Early Anglo-Saxon England', *Journal of Social Archaeology*, 13.2 (2013). DOI: 10.1177/1469605312469455.

Buchanan, Ashley, 'Plant of the Month: Dittany', *JStor Daily* (23 September 2020). https://daily.jstor.org/plant-of-the-month-dittany/ (accessed 13 July 2021).

Buck, R. A., 'Woman's Milk in Anglo-Saxon and Later Medieval Medical Texts', *Neophilologus*, 96.3 (2012), 467–85.

Bullough, Vern and Cameron Campbell, 'Female Longevity and Diet in the Middle Ages', *Speculum*, 55.2 (1980), 317–25.

Butler, Sara M., 'Abortion by Assault: Violence against Pregnant Women in Thirteenth- and Fourteenth-Century England', *Journal of Women's History*, 17.4 (2005), 9–31.

Buttery, Neil, 'On a Mushroom Hunt', *British Food: A History* (6 November 2012). https://britishfoodhistory.com/2012/11/06/on-the-hunt-for-mushrooms/ (accessed 28 March 2020).

Cameron, Angus, Ashley Crandell Amos, Antonette diPaolo Healey et al. (eds), *Dictionary of Old English: A to I Online* (Toronto: Dictionary of Old English Project, 2018). https://tapor.library.utoronto.ca/doe/ (accessed 23 December 2023).

Cameron, M. L., *Anglo-Saxon Medicine* (Cambridge: Cambridge University Press, 1993).

Cauterucci, Christina, 'Ignorance Is Blessed', *Slate* (15 May 2019), https://slate.com/news-and-politics/2019/05/alabama-abortion-law-republican-ignorance-female-reproduction.html (accessed 3 March 2020).

Cavell, Megan, *Weaving Words and Binding Bodies: The Poetics of Human Experience in Old English Literature* (Toronto: University of Toronto Press, 2016).

Cayton, H. M., 'Anglo-Saxon Medicine with Its Social Context', PhD thesis (Durham University, 1977).

CDC Newsroom, 'Racial and Ethnic Disparities Continue in Pregnancy-Related Death' (6 September 2019). www.cdc.gov/media/releases/2019/p0905-racial-ethnic-disparities-pregnancy-deaths.html (accessed 27 June 2023).

Center for Disease Control and Prevention, 'Stillbirth: Data and Statistics' (last reviewed 4 October 2022). www.cdc.gov/ncbddd/stillbirth/data.html (accessed 16 July 2023).

Chardonnens, L. S., *Anglo-Saxon Prognostics, 900–1100* (Leiden: Brill, 2007).

Clark Hall, J. R., *A Concise Anglo-Saxon Dictionary*, 4th edn (Cambridge: Cambridge University Press, 1960).

Cockayne, Thomas Oswald, *Leechdoms, wortcunning, and starcraft of early England. Being a collection of documents, for the most part never before printed, illustrating the history of science in this country before the Norman Conquest*, 3 vols (London: Longman, Green, Longman, Roberts and Green, 1864–66).

Cohen, David, 'Earlier. Akin: "Legitimate Rape" Rarely Leads to Pregnancy', *Politico* (19 August 2012). www.politico.com/story/2012/08/akin-legitimate-rape-victims-don't-get-pregnant-079864 (accessed 24 June 2022).

Cohen, David S., Greer Donley and Rachel Rebouché, 'The New Abortion Battleground', *Columbia Law Review*, 123.1 (January 2023), 1–100.

Cooper Owens, Deirdre, 'Listening to Black Women Saves Black Lives', *Lancet*, 397.10276 (27 February 2021), 788–9.

Crawford, Sally, *Childhood in Anglo-Saxon England* (Stroud: Sutton, 1999).

Criado Perez, Caroline, *Invisible Women: Data Bias in a World Designed for Men* (New York: Abrams Press, 2019).

Cross, J. E., *Two Old English Apocrypha and Their Manuscript Source: The 'Gospel of Nichodemus' and 'The Avenging of the Saviour'*, Cambridge Studies in Anglo-Saxon England 19 (Cambridge: Cambridge University Press, 1997).

Crow, Madison, Colleen Zori and Davide Zori, 'Doctrinal and Physical Marginality in Christian Death: The Burial of Unbaptized Infants in Medieval Italy', *Religions*, 11.12 (2020), 678.

Danielsson, Krissi, 'Complications after a Miscarriage', *Verywell Family*. www.verywellfamily.com/possible-complications-after-a-miscarriage-2371525 (accessed 3 June 2020).

Danielsson, Krissi, 'Making Sense of Miscarriage Statistics', *Verywell Family* (20 April 2020). www.verywellfamily.com/making-sense-of-miscarriage-statistics-2371721 (accessed 25 June 2021).

de Vogue, Ariane and Veronica Stracqualursi, 'Kavanaugh "Abortion-Inducing Drug" Comment Draws Scrutiny', CNN (7 September 2018). www.cnn.com/2018/09/07/politics/brett-kavanaugh-hearing-birth-control/index.html (accessed 6 July 2023).

De Vriend, Hubert Jan (ed.), *The Old English Herbarium and Medicina de Quadrupedibus*, Early English Text Society (Oxford: Oxford University Press, 1984).

DeVun, Leah, *The Shape of Sex: Nonbinary Gender from Genesis to the Renaissance* (New York: Columbia University Press, 2021).

diPaolo Healey, Antoinette, with John Price Wilkin and Xin Xiang (eds), *Dictionary of Old English Web Corpus* (Toronto: Dictionary of Old English Project, 2009). https://doe.artsci.utoronto.ca/?p=498 (accessed 23 December 2023).

Dockray-Miller, Mary, 'Breasts and Babies: The Maternal Body of Eve in the Junius 11 *Genesis*', in Benjamin Withers and Jonathan Wilcox (eds), *Naked before God* (Morgantown: West Virginia University Press, 2003), pp. 221–56.

Dockray-Miller, Mary, *Motherhood and Mothering in Anglo-Saxon England* (London: Palgrave Macmillan, 2000).

Doyle, Conan, 'Anglo-Saxon Medicine and Disease: A Semantic Approach', 2 vols, PhD thesis (University of Cambridge, 2017).

Ellis, Havelock, 'The Influence of Menstruation on the Position of Women', *Studies in the Psychology of Sex*, Vol. I, 3rd edn (Philadelphia, F. A. Davis, 1920).

England, Charlotte, 'Erectile Dysfunction Studies Outnumber PMS Research by Five to One', *Independent* (19 August 2016). www.independent.co.uk/news/science/pms-erectile-dysfunction-studies-penis-problems-period-pre-menstrual-pains-science-disparity-a7198681.html (accessed 13 February 2020).

Estes, Heide, 'Menstruation, Infirmity, and Religious Observance from Ecclesiastical History', in Cameron Hunt McNabb (ed.), *Medieval Disability Sourcebook* (Goleta, CA: Punctum Books, 2020), pp. 341–44.

Fell, Christine, with Cecily Clark and Elizabeth Williams, *Women in Anglo-Saxon England and the Impact of 1066* (London: British Museum Publications, 1984).

Filipovic, Jill, 'Alabama's Abortion Bill Is Immoral, Inhumane, and Wildly Inconsistent', *Vanity Fair* (15 May 2019). www.vanityfair.com/style/2019/05/alabamas-abortion-bill-is-immoral-inhumane-and-wildly-inconsistent (accessed 6 July 2023).

Flowers, Jennifer Elaine, 'The Journey of Young Souls in Early Medieval England (c. 850–c.1050)', DPhil thesis (University of Oxford, 2020).
Forbes, Scott, *A Natural History of Families* (Princeton: Princeton University Press, 2005).
Frank, Roberta, 'Sex in the Dictionary of Old English', in Mark Amodio and Katherine O'Brien O'Keeffe (eds), *Unlocking the Wordhord: Anglo-Saxon Studies in Memory of Edward B. Irving, Jr.* (Toronto: University of Toronto Press, 2003), pp. 302–12.
Frantzen, Allen (ed), *Anglo-Saxon Penitentials: A Cultural Database, Oxford, Bodleian Library, Junius 121, s. XI¾; Worcester, 93b. X14.07.01.* www.anglo-saxon.net/penance/index.php?p=JUNIUS_93b (accessed 16 July 2023).
Freidenfelds, Lara, *The Modern Period: Menstruation in Twentieth-Century America* (Baltimore: Johns Hopkins University Press, 2009).
Fulk, R. D. and Stefan Jurasinski (eds), *The Old English Canons of Theodore*, Early English Text Society (Oxford: Oxford University Press, 2012).
Garner, Lori Ann, *Hybrid Healing: Old English Remedies and Medical Texts* (Manchester: Manchester University Press, 2022).
Garver, Valerie, 'Childbearing and Infancy in the Carolingian World', *Journal of the History of Sexuality*, 21.2 (May 2012), 208–44.
Geake, Helen, 'The Use of Grave-Goods in Conversion Period England c. 600–c.850 A.D.', 2 vols, PhD thesis (University of York, 1995).
Genuinely Irish Old Moore's Almanac, The, 'The Mysterious and Lost Magic Mushroom Rituals of the Ancient Celts'. https://oldmooresalmanac.com/the-mysterious-and-lost-magic-mushroom-rituals-of-the-ancient-celts/# (accessed 28 March 2020).
Gilchrist, Roberta, *Sacred Heritage: Monastic Archeology, Identities, Beliefs* (Cambridge: Cambridge University Press, 2020).
Gowri, Vaidyanathan, 'Abortion and Ensoulment', *Sultan Qaboos University Medical Journal*, 13.1 (February 2013), 1–2.
Grattan, J. H. G. *Anglo-Saxon Magic and Medicine* (Oxford: Oxford University Press, 1952).
Graves, Rolande, *Born to Procreate: Women and Childbirth in France from the Middle Ages to the Eighteenth Century* (Pieterlen: Peter Lang, 2000).
Green, Monica, 'From "Diseases of Women" to "Secrets of Women": The Transformation of Gynecological Literature in the Later Middle Ages', *Journal of Medieval and Early Modern Studies*, 30.1 (2000), 5–39.
Green, Monica, 'Gendering the History of Women's Healthcare', *Gender & History*, 20.3 (2008), 487–518.
Green, Monica, *Making Women's Medicine Masculine: The Rise of Male Authority in Pre-Modern Gynaecology* (Oxford: Oxford University Press, 2008).
Green, Monica H. (ed. and trans.), *The Trotula: An English Translation of the Medieval Compendium of Women's Medicine* (Philadelphia: University of Pennsylvania Press, 2002).

Greenwood, Brad N., Seth Carnahan and Laura Huang, 'Patient–Physician Gender Concordance and Increased Mortality among Female Heart Attack Patients', *Proceedings of the National Academy of Sciences*, 115.34 (6 August 2018), 8569–74. DOI:10.1073/pnas.1800097115.

Gregory, Elizabeth C. W., Claudia P. Valenzuela and Donna L. Hoyert, 'Fetal Mortality: United States, 2020', *National Vital Statistics Reports*, 71.4 (4 August 2022), 1–19.

Grendon, Felix, 'The Anglo-Saxon Charms', *The Journal of American Folklore*, 22.84 (April–June 1909), 105–237.

Guo, Yifan, Na Zhang, Daoqiang Zhang et al., 'Iron Homeostasis in Pregnancy and Spontaneous Abortion', *American Journal of Hematology*, 94.2 (February 2019), 184–8. DOI: 10.1002/ajh.25341 (accessed 8 December 2021).

Gutt, Blake and Alicia Spencer-Hall, 'Introduction', in Blake Gutt and Alicia Spencer-Hall (eds), *Trans and Genderqueer Subjects in Medieval Hagiography* (Amsterdam: Amsterdam University Press, 2021), pp. 11–40.

Han, Christina and Cara C. Heuser, 'Antiabortion Heartbeat Bills Are Neither Morally nor Legally Sound', *Scientific American* (23 January 2023). www.scientificamerican.com/article/antiabortion-heartbeat-bills-are-neither-morally-nor-legally-sound/ (accessed 15 July 2023).

Hankins, Freda Richards, '*Bald's Leechbook* Reconsidered', PhD thesis (University of North Carolina Chapel Hill, 1992).

Harlow, Sioban D. and Oona M. R. Campbell, 'Menstrual Dysfunction: A Missed Opportunity for Improving Reproductive Health in Developing Countries', *Reproductive Health Matters*, 8.15 (May 2000), 142–7.

Harrington, Susanmarie, 'Women, Literacy, and Intellectual Culture in Anglo-Saxon England', PhD thesis (University of Michigan, 1990).

Hensley, Matthew, Melissa E. Bauer, Lindsay K. Admon and Hallie C. Prescott, 'Incidence of Maternal Sepsis and Sepsis-Related Maternal Deaths in the United States', *JAMA*, 322.890 (3 September 2019). DOI:10.1001/jama.2019.9818 (accessed 3 June 2020).

Holdcroft, Anita, 'Gender Bias in Research: How Does It Affect Evidence Based Medicine?', *Journal of the Royal Society of Medicine*, 100.1 (January 2007), 2–3. DOI: 10.1258/jrsm.100.1.2 (accessed 28 February 2020).

Holley, Peter and Dan Solomon, 'Your Questions about Texas's New Abortion Law, Answered', *Texas Monthly* (7 October 2021). www.texasmonthly.com/news-politics/texas-abortion-law-explained/ (accessed 10 December 2021).

Hollis, Stephanie, *Anglo-Saxon Women and the Church: Sharing a Common Fate* (Woodbridge: Boydell Press, 1992).

Horden, Peregrine, 'What's Wrong with Early Medieval Medicine?', *Social History of Medicine*, 24.1 (2009), 5–25.

In Our Own Voice: National Black Women's Reproductive Justice Agenda, 'Black Women and Reproductive Health'. http://blackrj.org/wp-content/uploads/2015/10/BlackWomen-andReproductiveHealthFS.pdf (accessed 27 June 2023).

Jolly, Karen, 'Part 1: Medieval Magic. Definitions, Beliefs, and Practices', in Karen Jolly, Catharina Raudvere, and Edward Peters (eds), *Witchcraft and Magic in Europe* (London: The Athlone Press, 2002), pp. 1–72.

Jolly, Karen, *Popular Religion in Late Saxon England: Elf Charms in Context* (Charlotte: University of North Carolina Press, 1996).

Jones, D. A., 'The Human Embryo in the Christian Tradition: A Reconsideration', *Journal of Medical Ethics*, 31 (2005), 710–13.

Jones, David Albert, 'Aquinas as an Advocate of Abortion? The Appeal to "Delayed Animation" in Contemporary Christian Ethical Debates on the Human Embryo', *Studies in Christian Ethics*, 26.1 (2013), 97–112.

Jones, Peter Murray and Lea T. Olsan, 'Performative Rituals for Conception and Childbirth in England, 900–1500', *Bulletin of the History of Medicine*, 89 (2015), 406–33.

Jurasinski, Stefan, *The Old English Penitentials and Anglo-Saxon Law* (Cambridge: Cambridge University Press, 2015).

Juynboll, G. H. A., 'Review of Basim F. Musallam, *Sex and Society in Islam: Birth Control before the Nineteenth Century*', *International Journal of Middle East Studies*, 18.4 (November 1986), 510–11.

Karras, Ruth Mazzo, *Sexuality in Medieval Europe: Doing unto Others* (London: Routledge, 2005).

Kenari, Hoorieh Mohammadi, Gholamreza Kordafshari, Maryam Moghimi, Fatemeh Eghbalian and Dariush Taher Khani, 'Review of Pharmacological Properties and Chemical Constituents of *Pastinaca sativa*', *Journal of Pharmacopuncture*, 24.1 (31 March 2021), 14–23.

Kesling, Emily, *Medical Texts in Anglo-Saxon Literary Culture* (Cambridge: D. S. Brewer, 2020).

Kesling, Emily, 'The Old English Medical Collections in the Literary Context', DPhil thesis (Oxford University, 2016).

KFF [Kaiser Family Foundation]. 'Abortion in the United States' (1 July 2022). www.kff.org/womens-health-policy/press-release/abortion-in-the-united-states/ (accessed 15 July 2023).

Khitamy, Badaway A. B., 'Divergent Views on Abortion and the Period of Ensoulment', *Sultan Qaboos University Medical Journal*, 13.1 (February 2013), 26–31.

Klein, Stacy S, 'Parenting and Childhood in the Fortunes of Men', in Susan Irvine and Winfried Rudolf (eds), *Childhood and Adolescence in Anglo-Saxon Literary Culture* (Toronto: University of Toronto Press, 2018), pp. 95–138.

Kontoyannis, Maria and Christos Katsetos, 'Midwives in Early Modern Europe (1400–1800)', *Health Science Journal*, 5.1 (2011), 32–6.

Lakin, Milton and Hadley Wood, 'Erectile Dysfunction', Cleveland Clinic Center for Continuing Education (2018). www.clevelandclinicmeded.com/medicalpubs/diseasemanagement/endocrinology/erectile-dysfunction (accessed 12 June 2023).

Laqueur, Thomas, *Making Sex: Body and Gender from the Greeks to Freud* (Cambridge, MA: Harvard University Press, 1990).

Learmonth, Imogen, 'The Gender Health Gap: Why Women's Bodies Shouldn't Be a Medical Mystery', Thred media (September 2020). https://thred.com/change/the-gender-health-gap-why-womens-bodies-shouldnt-be-a-medical-mystery/ (accessed 3 November 2021).

Lee, Becky R. 'The Purification of Women after Childbirth: A Window onto Medieval Perceptions of Women', *Florilegium*, 14 (1995–96), 43–55.

Lee, Christina, *Ancientbiotics*. https://ancientbiotics.co.uk/ (accessed 14 June 2023).

Lee, Christina, 'Threads and Needles: The Use of Textiles for Medical Purposes', in Maren Clegg Hyer and Jill Frederick (eds), *Textiles, Text, Intertext: Essays in Honour of Gale R. Owen-Crocker* (Woodbridge: Boydell Press, 2016), pp. 103–17.

Lees, Clare and Gillian Overing, *Double Agents: Women and Clerical Culture in Anglo-Saxon England* (Philadelphia: University of Pennsylvania Press, 2001).

Lev, Efraim and Zohar Amar, *Practical 'Materia Medica' of the Medieval Eastern Mediterranean According to the Cairo Genizah* (Leiden: Brill, 2008).

Liuzza, R. M., *Anglo-Saxon Prognostics: An Edition and Translation of Texts from London, British Library, MS Cotton Tiberius A.iii* (London: D. S. Brewer, 2011).

Lopata, Alex, 'History of the Egg in Embryology', *Journal of Mammalian Ova Research*, 26.1 (2009), 2–9.

Lucy, Sam and Andrew Reynolds (eds), *Burial in Early Medieval England and Wales* (Abingdon: Routledge, 2002).

Mandal, Ananya, 'Rosacea and Menopause', *NewsMedical Life Sciences* (20 January 2023). www.news-medical.net/health/Rosacea-and-Menopause.aspx (accessed 13 June 2023.

Mattern, Susan P., 'A Time of Change: A History of Our Understanding of the Menopause. How Has the Way in which We Understand the Menopause Evolved over Time?', *History Matters* (28 June 2021). www.historyextra.com/period/20th-century/a-time-of-change-understanding-menopause (accessed 6 June 2023).

Maude, Kathryn, *Addressing Women in Early Medieval Religious Texts* (Woodbridge: Boydell and Brewer, 2021).

Mayo Clinic, 'Hydrocele' (updated 12 January 2023), www.mayoclinic.org/diseases-conditions/hydrocele/symptoms-causes/syc-20363969 (accessed 8 July 2023).

Mazziotta, Julie, 'Texas Website where People Can Report Violators of Abortion Ban Shut Down a Second Time', *People* (7 September 2021). https://people.com/health/texas-site-to-report-violators-of-the-highly-restrictive-abortion-law-shut-down-a-second-time/ (accessed 10 December 2021).

Meaney, Audrey, *Anglo-Saxon Amulets and Curing Stones* (Oxford: British Archaeological Reports, 1981).

Meens, Rob, 'A Background to Augustine's Mission to Anglo-Saxon England', *Anglo-Saxon England*, 23 (1994), 5–17.
Menuge, Noel James, 'A Few Home Truths: The Medieval Mother as Guardian in Romance and Law', in Noel James Menuge (ed.), *Medieval Women and the Law* (Woodbridge: Boydell and Brewer, 2003).
Merone, Lea, Komla Tsey, Darren Russell and Cate Nagle, 'Sex Inequalities in Medical Research: A Systematic Scoping Review of the Literature', *Women's Health Reports*, 3.1 (2022), 49–59.
Miller, Richard J., 'Religion as a Product of Psychotropic Drug Use', *The Atlantic* (27 December 2013).
Mills, Robert, *Seeing Sodomy in the Middle Ages* (Chicago: University of Chicago Press, 2015).
Mistry, Zubin, *Abortion in the Early Middle Ages, c. 500–900* (Woodbridge: Boydell and Brewer, 2017).
Miyashiro, Adam, 'Decolonizing Anglo-Saxon Studies: A Response to ISAS in Honolulu', *In the Middle* (29 July 2017). www.inthemedievalmiddle.com/2017/07/decolonizing-anglo-saxon-studies.html (accessed 25 October 2021).
Miyashiro, Adam, '"Our Deeper Past": Race, Settler Colonialism, and Medieval Heritage Politics', *Literature Compass*, 16 (2019), 1–11.
Miyashiro, Adam, 'Race, White Supremacy, and the Middle Ages', conference presentation at International Congress on Medieval Studies, Western Michigan University, 13 May 2018.
Morus Londinium, 'Timeline of the Mulberry in London'. www.moruslondinium.org/research/timeline (accessed 30 July 2021).
Mosconi, Lisa, 'Exploring the Link between Menopause and Alzheimer's', *Medium* (30 May 2019). https://medium.com/neurotrack/menopause-and-alzheimers-1c455f29fe16 (accessed 3 November 2021).
Mosleh, Ghazaleh, Parmis Badr, Amir Azadi, Zohreh Abolhassanzadeh, Seyed Vahid Hosseini and Abdolali Mohagheghzadeh, 'Wallflower (*Erysimum cheiri* (L.) Crantz) from Past to Future', *Research Journal of Pharmacognosy*, 6.2 (2019), 85–95.
Musallam, Basim F., *Sex and Society in Islam: Birth Control before the Nineteenth Century* (Cambridge: Cambridge University Press, 1983).
Niles, John P. and Maria D'Aronco (eds and trans), *Anglo-Saxon Medical Texts*, Vol. I, *The Old English Herbal, Lacnunga, and Other Texts*, Dumbarton Oaks Medieval Library (Cambridge, MA: Harvard University Press, 2023).
Olsan, Lea T., 'Charms in Medieval Memory', in Jonathan Roper (ed.), *Charms and Charming in Europe* (London: Palgrave Macmillan, 2004), pp. 59–90.
Osborn, Marijane, 'Anglo-Saxon Ethnobotany: Women's Reproductive Medicine in *Leech Book III*', in Peter Dendl and Alaine Touwaide (eds), *Health and Healing from the Medieval Garden* (Woodbridge: Boydell, 2008), pp. 145–61.
Oswald, Dana, *Monsters, Gender, and Sexuality in Medieval English Literature* (Woodbridge: Boydell and Brewer, 2010).

Owen-Crocker, Gale R., 'Anglo-Saxon Women, Woman, and Womanhood', in Helene Scheck and Christine E. Kozikowski (eds), *New Readings on Women and Early Medieval English Literature and Culture: Cross-Disciplinary Studies in Honour of Helen Damico* (Amsterdam: Amsterdam University Press, 2019), pp. 23–41.

Payer, Pierre J., *Sex and the Penitentials: The Development of a Sexual Code 550–1150* (Toronto: University of Toronto Press, 1984).

PBS, 'How the U.S. Compares with the Rest of the World on Abortion Rights', *PBS News Hour* (1 July 2022). www.pbs.org/newshour/politics/how-the-u-s-compares-with-the-rest-of-the-world-on-abortion-rights (accessed 15 July 2023).

Pettit, Edward Thomas (ed. and trans.), *Anglo-Saxon Remedies, Charms, and Prayers from the British Library MS Harley 585: The Lacnunga*, 2 vols (Lewiston: Edwin Mellen Press, 2001).

Pettit, Edward Thomas (ed. and trans.), 'A Critical Edition of the Anglo-Saxon *Lacnunga* of BL MS Harley 585', PhD thesis (King's College London, 1996).

Pew Research Center, 'America's Abortion Quandary' (6 May 2022). www.pewresearch.org/religion/2022/05/06/americas-abortion-quandary/ (accessed 15 July 2023).

Pollington, Stephen, *Leechcraft: Early English Charms, Plantlore, and Healing* (Ely: Anglo-Saxon Books, 2000).

Pollycove, Ricki, Frederick Naftolin and James A. Simon, 'The Evolutionary Origin and Significance of Menopause', *Menopause*, 18.3 (2011), 336–42. DOI: 10.1097/gme.0b013e3181ed957a.

Pulsiano, Philip and Elaine Treharne (eds), *A Companion to Anglo-Saxon Literature* (London: Blackwell, 2017).

Raday, Frances and the Working Group on the Issue of Discrimination Against Women in Law and in Practice, 'Women's Autonomy, Equality and Reproductive Health in International Human Rights: Between Recognition, Backlash and Regressive Trends', *United Nations Human Rights Special Procedures* (October 2017). www.ohchr.org/WomensAutonomyEqualityReproductiveHealth.pdf (accessed 15 July 2023).

Rambaran-Olm, Mary, 'Anglo-Saxon Studies [Early English Studies], Academia and White Supremacy', *Medium* (27 June 2018). https://mrambaranolm.medium.com/anglo-saxon-studies-academia-and-white-supremacy-17c87b360bf3 (accessed 25 October 2021).

Rambaran-Olm, Mary, 'History Bites: Resources on the Problematic Term "Anglo-Saxon", Part 1', *Medium* (7 September 2020). https://mrambaranolm.medium.com/history-bites-resources-on-the-problematic-term-anglo-saxon-part-1–9320b6a09eb7 (accessed 25 April 2022).

Rambaran-Olm, Mary, 'History Bites: Resources on the Problematic Term "Anglo-Saxon", Part 3', *Medium* (7 September 2020). https://mrambaranolm.medium.com/history-bites-resources-on-the-problematic-term-anglo-saxon-part-3–2f38919569f0 (accessed 25 October 2021).

Rambaran-Olm, Mary, 'Misnaming the Medieval: Rejecting "Anglo-Saxon" Studies', *History Workshop* (4 November 2019). www.historyworkshop.org.uk/misnaming-the-medieval-rejecting-anglo-saxon-studies/ (accessed 25 October 2021).

Rambaran-Olm, Mary, with Erik Wade, 'The Many Myths of the Term "Anglo-Saxon"', *Smithsonian Magazine* (14 July 2021). www.smithsonianmag.com/history/many-myths-term-anglo-saxon-180978169/ (accessed 25 October 2021).

Rauer, Christine, '*Mann* and Gender in Old English Prose', *Neophilologus*, 131 (2017), 139–58.

Reimagining Policy: In Pursuit of Black Reproductive Justice, 2023 Black Reproductive Justice Policy Agenda. https://blackrj.org/blackrjpolicyagenda/ (accessed 27 June 2023).

Riccomi, Giulia, Cristina Felici and Valentina Giuffra, 'Maternal-Fetal Death in Medieval Pieve di Pava (Central Italy, 10th–12th Century AD)', *International Journal of Osteoarchaeology* 31.5 (2021), 701–15.

Riddle, John M., *Contraception and Abortion from the Ancient World to the Renaissance* (Cambridge, MA: Harvard University Press, 1994).

Riddle, John M., 'Contraception and Early Abortion in the Middle Ages', in Vern L. Bullough and James A. Brundage (eds), *Handbook of Medieval Sexuality* (New York: Garland, 1996), pp. 261–77.

Roberts, Jane, Christian Kay and Lynne Grundy, *A Thesaurus of Old English* (Leiden: Brill, 2000). https://oldenglishthesaurus.arts.gla.ac.uk/ (accessed 9 January 2018).

Romm, Aviva, *Botanical Medicine for Women's Health* (London: Churchill/Livingstone, 2010).

Rubin, Stanley, 'The Medical Practitioner in Anglo-Saxon England', *Journal of the Royal College of General Practitioners*, 20.97 (1970), 63–71.

Sayer, Duncan, 'Christian Burial Practice in the Early Middle Ages: Rethinking the Anglo-Saxon Funerary Sphere', *History Compass*, 11.2 (2013), 133–46.

Sayer, Duncan, 'Death and the Family: Developing a Generational Chronology', *Journal of Social Archaeology*, 10.1 (2010), 59–91.

Sayer, Duncan, '"Sons of Athelings Given to the Earth": Infant Mortality within Anglo-Saxon Mortuary Geography', *Medieval Archaeology*, 58.1 (2014), 78–103.

Sayer, Duncan and Sam D. Dickinson, 'Reconsidering Obstetric Death and Female Fertility in Anglo-Saxon England', *World Archaeology*, 45.2 (2013), 285–97.

Scragg, Donald, 'Old English in the Margins', in Maren Clegg Hyer and Jill Frederick (eds), *Textiles, Text, Intertext: Essays in Honour of Gale R. Owen-Crocker* (Woodbridge: Boydell, 2016), pp. 171–80.

Scragg, Donald, '*Wifcyppe* and the Cynewulf and Cyneheard Episode', in Jane Roberts, Janet L. Nelson and Malcolm Godden (eds), *Alfred the Wise* (Cambridge: D. S. Brewer, 1997), pp. 179–86.

Skeat, W. W., *The Four Gospels in Anglo-Saxon, Northumbrian, and Old Mercian Versions* (Cambridge: Cambridge University Press, 1871–87).

Slawson, Nicola. '"Women Have Been Woefully Neglected": Does Medical Science Have a Gender Problem?', *Guardian* (18 December 2019). www.theguardian.com/education/2019/dec/18/women-have-been-woefully-neglected-does-medical-science-have-a-gender-problem (accessed 3 November 2021).

Stafford, Pauline, *Queen Emma and Queen Edith: Queenship and Women's Power in Eleventh-Century England* (Hoboken, NJ: Wiley Blackwell, 2001).

Stein, Elissa and Susan Kim, *Flow: The Cultural History of Menstruation* (New York: St Martin's Griffin, 2009).

Steinbert, Jecca R., Brandon E. Turner, Brannon T. Weeks et al., 'Analysis of Female Enrollment and Participant Sex by Burden of Disease in US Clinical Trials between 2000 and 2020', *JAMA Network Open*, 4.6 (2021). DOI: 10.1001/jamanetworkopen.2021.13749.

Stoertz, Fiona Harris, 'Suffering and Survival in Medieval English Childbirth', in Cathy Jorgensen Itnyre (ed.), *Medieval Family Roles* (Hoboken, NJ: Garland Press, 1996), pp. 101–20.

Stoodley, N., 'Multiple Burials, Multiple Meanings? Interpreting the Early Anglo-Saxon Multiple Interment', in S. Lucy and A. Reynolds (eds), *Burial in Early Medieval England and Wales* (Leeds: Society for Medieval Archaeology, 2002), pp. 103–21.

Stoodley, N., *The Spindle and the Spear: A Critical Enquiry into the Construction and Meaning of Gender in the Early Anglo-Saxon Burial Rite*, British Archaeological Reports 288 (Oxford: BAR, 1999).

Sullivan, Sean, 'Todd Akin Takes Back Apology for "Legitimate Rape" Comment', *Washington Post* (10 July 2014). www.washingtonpost.com/news/post-politics/wp/2014/07/10/todd-akin-takes-back-apology-for-legitimate-rape-comment/ (accessed 6 July 2023).

Swan, Mary, 'Remembering Veronica in Anglo-Saxon England', in Elaine Treharne (ed.), *Writing Gender and Genre in Medieval Literature* (London: D. S. Brewer, 2002), pp. 19–40.

Sweany, Erin, 'Unsettling Comparisons: Ethical Considerations of Comparative Approaches to the Old English Medical Corpus', *English Language Notes*, 58.2 (October 2020), 83–100.

Thompson, Victoria, *Death and Dying in Anglo-Saxon England* (Woodbridge: Boydell, 2004).

Traves, Alex, 'Genealogy and Royal Women in Asser's Life of King Alfred: Politics, Prestige, and Maternal Kinship in Early Medieval England', *Early Medieval Europe*, 30.1 (2022), 101–24.

Tyszka, Przemysław, 'The Conceptualisation of Men and Women by the Authors of Penitentials', in Anndrzej Pleszczynski, Joanna Sobiesiak, Michał Tomaszek and Przemysław Tyszka (eds), *Imagined Communities: Constructing Collective Identities in Medieval Europe* (Leiden: Brill, 2018), pp. 222–43.

UN News, 'Break Taboo around Menstruation, Act to End "disempowering" Discrimination, Say UN Experts' (5 March 2019).

https://news.un.org/en/story/2019/03/1034131#:~:text=A%20group%20of%20seven%20United,to%20end%20%E2%80%9Cdisempowering%E2%80%9D%20discrimination (accessed 25 July 2022).

United Nations Population Fund, 'Menstruation and Human Rights – Frequently Asked Questions' (May 2022). www.unfpa.org/menstruationfaq (accessed 25 July 2022).

Van Arsdall, Anne, *Medieval Herbal Remedies: The Old English Herbarium and Anglo-Saxon Medicine* (London: Routledge, 2022).

Veritas-Certum, 'The Ishango Bone: A 22,000-Year-Old Lunar Calendar Made by Women as the First Mathematicians'. www.reddit.com/r/badhistory/comments/m5hzjw/the_ishango_bone_a_22000_year_old_lunar_calendar/ (accessed 6 July 2023).

Villarosa, Linda, 'Why America's Black Mothers and Babies Are in a Life-or-Death Crisis', *New York Times Magazine* (11 April 2018). www.nytimes.com/2018/04/11/magazine/black-mothers-babies-death-maternal-mortality.html (accessed 31 May 2018).

Voth, Christine, 'An Analysis of the Tenth-Century Anglo-Saxon Manuscript London, British Library, Royal 12.D.xvii, PhD thesis (University of Cambridge, 2015).

Voth, Christine, 'Women and "Women's Medicine", Early Medieval England: From Text to Practice', in R. Trilling, R. Norris and R. Stephenson (eds), *Feminist Approaches to Anglo-Saxon Studies* (Amsterdam: Amsterdam University Press, 2023), pp. 279–316.

Wade, Erik, '*Pater* Don't Preach: Byzantine Theology, Female Sexuality, and Histories of Global Encounter in the "English" *Pænitentiale Theodori*', *The Medieval Globe*, 4.2 (2018), 1–28.

Wald, Anna, 'Comment: When Postpartum Maternal Sepsis Is Fatal', *NEJM Journal Watch* (23 September 2019). www.jwatch.org/na49866/2019/09/23/when-postpartum-maternal-sepsis-fatal (accessed 3 June 2020).

Weston, L. M. C., 'Women's Medicine, Women's Magic', *Modern Philology*, 92.3 (1995), 279–93.

Williams, Timothy, 'New Abortion Bills Are So Tough that Some Conservatives Have Qualms', *New York Times* (4 December 2019). www.nytimes.com/2019/12/04/us/abortion-bills-ohio-ectopic-pregnancy.html (accessed 6 July 2023).

Wilson, Adrian, *The Making of Man-Midwifery: Childbirth in England 1660–1770* (Cambridge, MA: Harvard University Press, 1995).

Włodarczak-Semczuk, Anna and Kacper Pempel, 'Death of Pregnant Woman Ignites debate about Abortion ban in Poland', Reuters (6 November 2021). www.reuters.com/world/europe/death-pregnant-woman-ignites-debate-about-abortion-ban-poland-2021-11-05/ (accessed 10 December 2021).

Wood, Charles T., 'The Doctors' Dilemma: Sin, Salvation, and the Menstrual Cycle in Medieval Thought', *Speculum: A Journal of Medieval Studies*, 56.4 (1981), 710–27.

Wootton, David, *Bad Medicine: Doctors Doing Harm since Hippocrates* (Oxford: Oxford University Press, 2007).
World Carrot Museum, 'Carrots and Their Contraceptive Properties', www.carrotmuseum.co.uk/cont.html (accessed 9 August 2022).
Wright, C. E. and Randolph Quirk (eds), *Bald's Leechbook (British Museum Royal Manuscript 12. D. xvii)*, Early English Manuscript Facsimiles 5 (Copenhagen: Rosenkilde and Bagger, 1955).
Wright, Michael, 'Anglo-Saxon Midwives', *ANQ: A Quarterly Journal of Short Articles, Notes and Reviews*, 11.1 (1998), 3–5.
Zacher, Samantha, *Preaching the Converted: The Style and Rhetoric of the Vercelli Book Homilies* (Toronto: University of Toronto Press, 2009).
Zacher, Samantha, 'The Source of Vercelli VII: An Address to Women', in Samantha Zacher and Andy Orchard (eds), *New Readings in the Vercelli Book* (Toronto: University of Toronto Press, 2009), pp. 98–149.
Zaslavsky, Claudia, 'Women as the First Mathematicians', *Newsletter of the International Study Group of Ethnomathematics*, 7.1 (1992), 1.

Index

abjection 9, 21, 49, 66, 77, 113, 129, 162
abortifacient 51–5, 65, 122, 133, 143–7, 156–7
abortion 2, 51–4, 66, 68–70, 82, 96, 137–9, 145–7, 151–62, 178, 184, 186–7
absolution 35
acenned 118–24
adl 37–42, 59, 85, 150, 184
aðl see adl
Ælfric 83, 98, 101, 102, 123, 167, 174
æþme 48
æwyrpan 154–6
afedan 92, 105–14, 124, 129
afeormian 21, 139–41, 151–8, 162
agency 2, 20–1, 33–4, 70–5, 79–81, 85, 91–5
amenorrhea 52, 154
Anglo-Saxon Dictionary (Bosworth–Toller) 15, 129
archaeology 10, 12–13, 20, 110
Aristotle 69, 95, 159, 169
astyrian 51–3, 145, 157
Augustine of Canterbury, St 37, 38, 40–2
authority 21, 33–4, 50, 73, 80, 86–7, 90–2, 140, 158–62, 171

Bald's Leechbook 4–5, 7–8, 126, 148, 151, 175, 176
'Table of Contents' 3, 8, 125, 127, 150
Banham, Debby *see* Voth, Christine, with Debby Banham
bath *see* bathing
bathing 54–5, 67, 68, 76–9, 115, 121, 146, 153
Bede 37–42, 173
beorþor 49, 105
beorþorþinen 6
binding 47–8, 63, 73–4, 116–19, 124–7
birth lunaria 72, 80–1, 86, 119
Black women 18
blodryne 37–8, 42, 53
blodsihtan 53, 150
blood 2, 37–8, 39–40, 42–3, 44–5, 49–50, 52, 69, 84, 129, 143, 149, 182, 185
British Museum 172
Broadstairs Woman 171–4
brooklime 54, 66, 144

calendar 68–9, 80, 93, 158–60
carrot 121, 122, 153
cennan 21, 75, 87–8, 105, 117–25
childbirth 1–2, 7, 10–20, 21, 39, 82–6, 104–9, 116–24, 141, 151–4, 158, 178–87

Index

clænsian 21, 74, 139–41, 147–52, 162
cleansing 20, 21, 39–40, 52–3, 74, 139–40, 147–53, 184, 186
Cockayne, Thomas Oswald 15, 24, 38, 84, 105, 125, 177
comfrey 63
community 7, 56, 91–4, 161, 178
conception 1, 19, 50–5, 69–95, 105–11, 113–22, 124, 126–8, 137–42, 146, 147, 151, 153, 155–60, 162, 178, 185–7
   of androgynous children 74–5, 120
   of female children 75–80, 87–8, 115–16, 117–19
   of male children 76, 87–8, 115–19
cwican 83, 92, 109–10
cwiþan 152–3

D&C *see* dilatation and curettage
deadboren 53, 139, 142–6, 162
death 10–13, 19, 81, 104, 155, 181
deer 73–4, 116, 181–2
DeVun, Leah 14
diagnostic body 20, 32–6
Dickinson, Sam D. *see* Sayer, Duncan and Sam D. Dickinson
Dictionary of Old English 16, 29, 38, 39, 43, 45, 65, 105, 114, 124, 129, 130, 133, 134, 147, 155, 183
diet 10, 180
dilatation and curettage (D&C) 141
disability 38–9, 72, 77, 90, 103
dittany 144–6
Dockray-Miller, Mary 120, 123, 173
DOE Web Corpus 8, 28, 44, 58, 59, 61, 99, 100, 102, 107, 165, 167, 168, 177

Early English Text Society 15
effacement 9–15, 16–21, 172
efficacy 1, 4, 66, 152
embryo 69, 72, 138, 143, 159
embryology 80–6, 100–1
emmenagogue 51, 66, 143–7, 154, 155–8
ensoulment 72, 82, 115, 140, 158–61
erectile dysfunction 18, 56, 181
euphemistic language 33, 43, 44, 143, 183–4

fertility 1, 13, 19–21, 34, 44, 47, 49, 50–2, 55–6, 68–80, 89–95, 97–8, 105–10, 156–8, 162, 171–3, 178, 182, 184–6
fleabane 122, 134
flewsan 37–8, 43, 44–50, 53, 63, 128
forlætan 52, 65
forstanden 43–4, 51, 54, 66, 105

Galen 5, 14, 28, 69–71, 95
geberan 21, 105–8, 124–8, 129, 134, 150
gecigde 51–2
gecynd 13, 37, 41–4, 47–9, 54, 62, 68, 78, 82, 145, 150
gecyndlim 13, 66
geeacnian 21, 73, 76–7, 79–80, 105–8, 114–19, 121, 129, 132, 133
gefedan 21, 130, 135
gefremman 122–3, 134, 181
gender binary 9–14, 127–8
   see also male; *mann*; *wif*; woman
genealogies 173–4, 188
Genesis 120, 123, 130
genitals 13, 43, 44, 47, 48, 49, 50, 51, 53, 66, 117, 118, 122, 124, 129, 145, 150, 151, 152, 179, 183, 186

gestation 70, 92, 105, 110, 114, 124, 166
gestational age 69, 70
gewrið 47, 48, 63, 64, 74, 116
graves 10–12, 15, 91–3, 104, 109–11, 113, 136, 172–3, 187–8
  see also *Lacnunga*, stepping-over-the-grave remedy
Green, Monica 4, 6–7, 50, 66, 155–7
Gregory, Pope 37–42, 61
grief 109–14
gynaecological concerns 1, 7, 15, 18, 49, 55, 152, 153, 162, 183, 184, 186

haemorrhage 12, 38, 42, 50, 65, 151, 185
hare 76–7, 120, 132
healers 6, 24
healing 5, 20, 36, 38, 79, 109, 114, 121, 122, 142–3, 150, 183
health 7, 14, 17, 18, 19, 32, 34, 37, 45, 55–6, 78–9, 93, 104, 137, 138, 141, 143, 145, 153, 174, 179
heartbeat 82
  heartbeat laws 137–8, 160
Hippocrates 69, 71
hormones 180, 183
hræpe 73, 100, 116
humoral medicine 46, 48–52, 55, 60, 63
husband 35, 60, 91–4, 98, 109, 114
hydrocele 90
hysteric philology 1–2, 14–20, 184

incantations 20, 93, 127
Indigenous women 17–18
infant loss 11, 108–14, 160–1, 162
infertility 1, 19, 73–80, 91–5, 97, 110
innoðe 13, 82, 117, 142, 143, 144
Ishango bone 68
Izabela 137–8, 162

Kesling, Emily 5–6, 7, 155–8

Lacnunga 4–5, 8, 91–4, 109–14, 125–7, 184
  milk remedy 111–13
  stepping-over-the-grave remedy 91–3, 109
  wool remedy 110–11
lactation 12, 131, 135, 164
Latin (tradition and language) 5–6, 13, 15, 24, 28, 33, 38, 39, 41, 44, 48, 59, 61, 63–4, 96, 100, 101, 105, 125–7, 129, 132, 135, 168, 182, 185
lawcodes 29, 61, 82, 124
Lee, Christina 111
Leechbook III 2, 4–5, 8, 22, 24, 43–4, 49, 54–5, 61, 65, 66, 105, 118–19, 121–3, 134, 143–7, 175–6
  brooklime and bath (38.1) 54, 66
  brooklime and pennyroyal (37.4) 143
  coriander see *Leechbook III*, henbane/coriander
  goosegrass (37.6) 49
  henbane/coriander (37.2) 118, 121
  smoking manure (38.2) 49
  wild carrot (37.1) 118, 121
Liuzza, Roy 71, 84, 90

male 11, 60, 61, 69, 75–7, 115, 155, 159, 172
  author 27
  body 14, 17–18, 28, 89–90, 174–8, 181, 186
  practitioner 6–7, 20–1, 25, 33, 72, 74, 82, 94–5, 102, 109
mann 14, 174–8, 188
manuscripts
  Bodleian Library, MS Hatton 76 24
  British Library, MS Cotton Vitellius A.iii 80

British Library, MS Cotton
    Vitellius C.iii 24, 26
British Library, MS Harley 585
    5, 130, 135
British Library, MS Harley
    6258b 24, 26
British Library, MS Royal 12.
    D.xvii 5
Meaney, Audrey 171–3
meat 76–8, 89–90, 111–13, 148
medical research, inequality in
    18, 178–81
Medicina de Quadrupedibus
    (OEM) 5, 8, 26, 28, 38,
    52–3, 73, 74–80, 115–16,
    120, 142–3, 148–50,
    167, 181–4
  boar gall (9.8) 134, 181
  bull testicles (12.14) 181
  deer antler (2.4) 182
  dear antler (3.1) 182
  deer antler (3.7) 182
  deer faeces (3.14) 181
  deer heart/womb (3.16)
    73, 116
  deer testicles (3.13) 181
  deer womb *see* deer heart/womb
  fox (4.1) 182
  goat gall (6.11) 8, 181
  hare stomach (5.14) 116
  hare testicle (5.13) 74, 128
  hare womb (5.12) 75, 120
  mulberry (2.3) 52
  mulberry (2.4) 128
  wolf milk (10.7) 142
menopause 31, 52, 178–86
menorrhagia 46, 185
menstruation 1–2, 18–21, 32,
    68–70, 74, 116, 126,
    139, 140, 143–60, 178,
    182, 184–7
midwives 6–7, 19, 160
milk 8, 49, 112–14, 121, 144, 177
  wolf 142, 157, 161
miscarriage 2, 74, 83, 93, 108–14,
    125, 127, 137–47, 152–8,
    160–2, 178, 184, 186

Miyashiro, Adam 15, 25
monaðadl 37, 38, 40–2
monaðgecynd 37, 42–4, 52–5, 105
monks 5–6, 54
monoðlican 37, 43, 44, 52, 53–4,
    64, 157
mortality 10–13, 141, 179–80
mulberry 148–50, 157, 161
mushrooms 75–80, 115

nettle 8
'Note on the Growth of the Fetus, A'
    72, 81–6
nutrition 10, 17, 46, 52, 68, 70,
    88, 161
nuts (as food) 88–9

obstetrics 3, 24, 97
Old English Herbarium (OEH)
    4–5, 8, 44–8, 52–5, 100,
    117–19, 121–4, 134
  bishop's weed (164.1) 52
  comfrey (menstrual) (60.1) 47
  comfrey (menstrual) (128.1) 47
  coriander (104.2) 117–18
  dittany (63.1) 144–5
  eryngo (173.1) 64
  fleabane/spikenard
    (143.2) 152–3
  fleabane/spikenard (143.3) 122
  German iris (158.2) 52
  nettle (178.6) 47–8
  parsnip *see Old English
    Herbarium* (OEH), wild
    carrot/parsnip
  pennyroyal (94.6) 143
  shepherd's purse (150.1) 52
  spikenard *see Old English
    Herbarium* (OEH), fleabane/
    spikenard
  St John's wort (152.2) 52
  wallflower (165.4) 53, 145–7
  wild carrot/parsnip (82.1)
    121, 122
  wild carrot/parsnip (82.2)
    153–4
  yarrow (175.2) 47

'Omens in Pregnancy, The' 72, 86–95, 102
ordinary bodies (vs extraordinary) 1–4, 7, 8–14, 20, 27, 33, 36, 42, 44, 157, 173, 184, 186
ovulation 69
Owen-Crocker, Gale 10, 12

parsnip 121, 153–4
partner (male) 40, 74–6, 79, 91–4, 109
partus preparator 152–3
penis 13, 28, 30, 134
penitentials 32–45, 50, 56, 82, 147, 154–5, 160–1, 162
pennyroyal 2, 143–7, 157, 165
Peri Didaxeon 99
Pettit, Edward Thomas 130
philology 1–2, 14–17, 29, 184
physician 6–7, 18, 34, 51, 55, 68, 91, 109, 137–8, 148, 161, 175–9, 185
pine tar 182–3, 191
Pliny 5, 133
prayer 20, 97, 126, 150
pregnancy 1–2, 11–12, 17, 20–1, 51–6, 68–95, 104–16, 124–7, 137–47, 152–62, 179, 184–7
prognostics 1, 21, 27, 70–95, 97, 119–20, 159, 185
purging 2, 21, 52, 74, 122, 137–62, 184

quickening 70–2, 83–6, 91–3, 109–14

Rambaran-Olm, Mary 15
reproduction 1–2, 12–14, 17–21, 44–7, 50, 53–6, 70, 74, 76, 80, 81–95, 104–28, 137–47, 151–62, 177–80, 186–7
reproductive complications 8, 17, 104, 179, 187
Reproductive Justice 17–18
Riddle, John M. 65, 96, 143, 155–8, 160, 169

Ride, Sally 32
ritual 38–42, 52, 59, 60, 73, 74, 93, 109, 110–14, 126–7, 131, 140, 147–51, 166
impurity 38–45, 60, 140, 148–50, 151
uncleanness 39, 147, 149

Sayer, Duncan and Sam D. Dickinson 10–13, 20, 179–80
Scriftboc 154–5
sexual acts 57, 60, 61, 181
sexual intercourse 8, 39, 40, 59, 69, 75–8, 97, 98, 107, 115
abstention from 33
prohibition of 39, 40, 61, 98
sexual pleasure 26
sin 33, 35, 39, 60
sinners *see* sin
skeletal remains 10–13, 179–80
smearing 48, 77–9, 100, 134
spikenard 122, 152–3
spontaneous abortion 146, 154
stillbirth 2, 53, 125, 137–62, 163, 166, 186
stirring (menstruation) 51–4, 64, 145, 158
Sweany, Erin 4, 189

tampons 32
testicles 74, 90, 128, 134, 181
Texas 70, 137, 138, 162
Texas Senate Bill 8 138
þrowian 41, 182
time 21, 39–40, 44–5, 51, 52, 54–5, 68–95, 97, 112, 115, 151, 156–62, 185–6
translators 1, 2, 5–6, 19–21, 33–4, 37–9, 41, 47, 56, 66, 84–5, 103, 107, 108, 111–13, 117, 120–8, 157, 176, 186
nineteenth century 15–16, 104–5, 128
tudder 53–4, 139–47, 162, 165
tudor see tudder

Index

United Nations 32
uterus 13, 18, 69, 70, 107, 113, 141, 153–4, 160, 169

vagina 13, 39, 146, 183
Van Arsdall, Anne 5, 47, 122
Vercelli Homilies 43, 77–9
Veronica 37–8, 42, 185
virility 181
Voth, Christine 3–4, 8, 182
 with Debby Banham 125
vulva 13, 173, 188

Wade, Erik 35–6, 60
wætan 48–50, 182
wætere 112, 113, 144, 152, 153, 175, 182

wallflower 145–7
wamb 13, 27, 148
wergild 87
wif 8–9
wild carrot *see* carrot; *Old English Herbarium* (OEH), wild carrot/parsnip
witleas 83–6, 101
woman
 category of x, 14, 127–8, 174–8
 women's afflictions 41–2, 149, 182, 183
womb 13–14, 53, 54, 73, 75, 82, 83, 88, 93, 108, 113, 114, 116, 119, 120, 124, 139, 143, 144, 150–8, 182, 186

EU authorised representative for GPSR:
Easy Access System Europe, Mustamäe tee 50,
10621 Tallinn, Estonia
gpsr.requests@easproject.com

www.ingramcontent.com/pod-product-compliance
Ingram Content Group UK Ltd.
Pitfield, Milton Keynes, MK11 3LW, UK
UKHW021830210426
5322IPUK00004B/126